PHYSICAL THERAPY
of the
GERIATRIC PATIENT

CLINICS IN PHYSICAL THERAPY
VOLUME 3

PHYSICAL THERAPY
of the
GERIATRIC PATIENT

Edited by

Osa Jackson, Ph.D., R.P.T.

Consultant, Norwegian Gerontological Institute;
Lecturer, Diakonissehusets Gerontological
Nursing Program, Oslo, Norway

CHURCHILL LIVINGSTONE

NEW YORK, EDINBURGH, LONDON, AND MELBOURNE

1983

© Churchill Livingstone Inc. 1983

Distributed in the United Kingdom by Churchill Livingstone, Robert Stevenson House, 1-3 Baxter's Place, Leith Walk, Edinburgh EH1 3AF and by associated companies, branches and representatives throughout the world.

First published 1983
Printed in U.S.A.

ISBN 0-443-08226-X
7   6   5   4   3   2   1

Library of Congress Cataloging in Publication Data
Main entry under title:

Physical therapy of the geriatric patient.

   (Clinics in physical therapy; v. 3)
   Bibliography: p.
   Includes index.
   1. Aged—Rehabilitation—Addresses, essays, lectures.
2. Physical therapy—Addresses, essays, lectures.
I. Jackson, Osa.   II. Series.   [DNLM: 1. Physical
therapy—In old age.   2. Rehabilitation—In old age.
W1 CL831CN v. 3 / WT 100 P578]
RC953.5.P48   1983   615.8′2′0880565   83-6624
ISBN 0-443-08226-X

Manufactured in the United States of America

Contributors

Louis R. Amundsen, R.P.T., Ph.D.
Director of Graduate Studies, Course in Physical Therapy, Department of Physical Medicine and Rehabilitation, University of Minnesota, Minneapolis, Minnesota

Louvain G. Arndts, O.T.R., M.P.H.
Assistant Professor, Course in Occupational Therapy, Department of Physical Medicine and Rehabilitation, University of Minnesota, Minneapolis, Minnesota

Carl I. Brahce, Ph.D.
Associate Research Scientist, Institute of Gerontology, The University of Michigan/Wayne State University, Ann Arbor, Michigan

Dennis J. Chapron, M.S.
Associate Clinical Professor, School of Pharmacy, University of Connecticut, Storrs, Connecticut; Assistant Director Pharmacokinetics Laboratory, University of Connecticut Health Center, Farmington, Connecticut

Marian L. Eliason, O.T.R., B.S.
Assistant Professor, Course in Occupational Therapy, Department of Physical Medicine and Rehabilitation, University of Minnesota, Minneapolis, Minnesota

Corinne T. Ellingham, R.P.T., M.S.
Assistant Professor, Course in Physical Therapy, Department of Physical Medicine and Rehabilitation, University of Minnesota, Minneapolis, Minnesota

Sue R. Hardy, O.T.R.
Staff Occupational Therapist, Maryland General Hospital, Baltimore, Maryland

Masayoshi Itoh, M.D., M.P.H.
Associate Professor of Clinical Rehabilitation Medicine, New York University School of Medicine; Associate Director, Department of Rehabilitation Medicine, Goldwater Memorial Hospital, New York University Medical Center, New York, New York

Osa Jackson, Ph.D., R.P.T.
Consultant, Norwegian Gerontological Institute; Lecturer, Diakonissehusets Gerontological Nursing Program, Oslo, Norway

Rosalie H. Lang, M.A.
Vice President, The Assistance Group for Human Resources Development, Storrs, Connecticut

Mathew H.M. Lee, M.D., M.P.H.
Professor of Clinical Rehabilitation Medicine and Clinical Professor of Oral and Maxillofacial Surgery, Clinical Professor of Behavioral Sciences and Community Health, Schools of Medicine and Dentistry, New York University; Director, Department of Rehabilitation Medicine, Goldwater Memorial Hospital, New York University Medical Center, New York, New York

Nancy L. Mace, M.A.
Assistant in Psychiatry and Coordinator, T. Rowe and Eleanor Price Teaching Service, Johns Hopkins University, Baltimore, Maryland

Rosemary A. Orgren, Ph.D.
Andrus Gerontology Center, University of Southern California, Los Angeles, California

David A. Peterson, Ph.D.
Andrus Gerontology Center, University of Southern California, Los Angeles, California

Barrie Pickles, B.P.T., M.S., M.C.S.P., M.C.P.A.
Associate Dean and Director, School of Rehabilitation Therapy, Faculty of Medicine, Queen's University, Kingston, Ontario

Peter V. Rabins, M.D., M.P.H.
Assistant Professor of Psychiatry and Director, T. Rowe and Eleanor Price Teaching Service, Johns Hopkins University, Baltimore, Maryland

Kenneth Solomon, M.D.
Associate Director for Education and Planning, Levindale Hebrew Geriatric Center and Hospital; Adjunct Assistant Professor, Department of Psychiatry, University of Maryland School of Medicine, Baltimore, Maryland

Preface

The need for a single source that would cover the basic concepts and principles of geriatric rehabilitation has been apparent to me whenever I teach undergraduates, advanced-degree students, and continuing-education participants. Geriatric rehabilitation is by necessity a team process where every member of the team must work from the foundation concepts of gerontology. This book is designed to provide a single source for the basic applied science of normal aging, common medical and functional problems among the elderly, and implications for therapeutic intervention.

In the past 30 years there has been an enormous increase in the number of persons over the age of 65. The field of rehabilitation and the profession of physical therapy were developed to treat a population commonly under the age of 65 and suffering from acute disease, trauma, polio, or war injuries. The treatment approaches, such as proprioceptive neuromuscular facilitation, Brunnstrom, etc., were developed and refined when the patient over age 70 was uncommon and not considered a candidate for rehabilitation.

In the 1980s the majority of patients seen in the hospital setting are over 55; the average age of nursing home patients is 80 or higher. The number of persons over the age of 65 is projected to continue to increase for the next 30 years. With these figures in mind, this text was developed to examine the unique changes in physiology/psychology/sociology/environmental adaptation that are commonly seen in advanced age. The content is meant to be relatively comprehensive, but there has not been an attempt to provide a forum for original research.

Chapter 1 provides the framework of reality for the book by examining the demographics of the aged population and the common multiple chronic degenerative medical problems of these patients. The implications of the changing demographics on the structure and process of rehabilitation for the aged is disscussed.

Chapter 2 is organized and written for optimal use by the undergraduate student and the practicing therapist. The chapter is organized with the presumption that the reader has a working knowledge of normal physiology. To help the reader, a brief review is made of those aspects of normal physiology which are commonly altered with advanced age. The reader is then presented with a description of the most relevant physiologic changes seen in advanced aging and the implications of these changes for clinical intervention. The review of physiology of aging is limited to the major body systems influenced by rehabilitation and physical therapy (connective tissue, bone, muscle, nerve, hormone).

Chapters 3, 4, and 5 present an overview of normal cognitive function in older adults and alterations due to psychological dysfunction. First, a presentation is made of older adult learning styles and how they differ from the way younger persons learn new psychomotor and cognitive skills. Second, the rationale for and the specific modifications necessary in clinical assessment in the presence of normal and common abnormal psychological changes with aging are reviewed. Lastly, the most common psychological dysfunctions seen in the elderly which can interfere with a positive rehabilitation outcome (depression, Alzheimer's, pseudodementia) are discussed. Chapter 5 focuses on the supportive intervention strategies and environmental manipulation that can be used by the rehabilitation team and the patient's family to promote effective participation of the patient in a personal rehabilitation program.

In advanced aging the body has an altered ability to metabolize medication; Chapter 6 presents a description of this physiological change. The common side effects of drug therapy (symptomatic postural hypotension, fatigue, weakness, depression, confusion, involuntary movements, dizziness, vertigo, ataxia, bowel and bladder incontinence) that can present obstacles to successful rehabilitation of the elderly are reviewed. The chapter is written to help the clinician screen out symptoms created by medication (which can usually be managed by adjustment in medication dosage, route, timing, etc.) and in this way allow maximum time and energy to be focused on treatment of the actual underlying disorders.

Chapter 7 examines the unique vulnerability of the emotional resources available to the average elderly patient. The common patterns of interaction among patient, family, meaningful others, and acquaintances during acute and prolonged illness are discussed. The chapter describes examples of family orientation and education programs that promote positive rehabilitation outcomes for the patient and his or her meaningful others.

Chapter 8 is a discussion of the clinical impact of the age related changes in the cardiopulmonary system. The chapter discusses the potential of the aging patient to participate in and benefit from exercise training. Emphasis is placed on the areas of needed modification in the basic process of exercise training if the training is to yield maximal results with the older patient.

Chapter 9 is an attempt to bring all the theory into practice. What are the normative functional changes seen in the elderly who are now 65–74, 75–84, and over 85 years of age and living in the community? What are the most common functional problems noted in each age category? In light of the functional status of healthy elderly, is it possible to screen for elderly at risk of institutionalization based on deterioration in ability to perform functional skills? How do we evaluate the older patient who presents with major acute and chronic problems in light of the normal functional problems commonly encountered in these age groups? Two sample assessment approaches are presented, one for use by the rehabilitation team as an approach to organizing care of the elderly and one for the detailed assessment of functional skills.

The goal of this text is to help the student and the clinician concretely examine current rehabilitation and physical therapy practices and to answer the question, Why must we modify or change these practices in order to achieve effective rehabilitation of the older patient? It is hoped that the text will be a catalyst in the evolution of a new goal for rehabilitation care—"independent living." The issue of independent living as a valid goal for rehabilitation intervention is under study by the United States Rehabilitation Services Administration. The statistics show that one in three elderly can be considered functionally disabled; thus this redefinition of the outcome of rehabilitation is timely.

I am deeply grateful to Dr. Otto Payton for giving me the opportunity to put this volume together and to the contributors for their practical insights. At this point an acknowledgement must also go to Dr. Moshe Feldenkrais, who has through his understanding of the human spirit and neurophysiology helped me to organize my thinking about the rehabilitation and physical therapy approaches that are needed if we are to be truly supportive of each individual in efforts to reach his or her personal potential.

I hope that this text will catalyze a close scrutiny of all rehabilitation and physical therapy practices to be sure that they are truly supportive of the goals of independent living rehabilitation for the elderly patient (see definition, Chapter 9). Up until now rehabilitation of the elderly has not consistently shown positive statistics for outcome. It is my fervent belief that if the foundation concepts of gerontology are used to develop a structure and process of rehabilitation and physical therapy care that is sensitive to the unique physiology, psychology, and sociology of aging, then independent living rehabilitation is a realistic goal for the majority of persons between the ages of 65 and 105.

Osa Jackson Klykken, Ph.D., R.P.T.

Contents

PHYSICAL THERAPY
of the
GERIATRIC PATIENT

1 | Rehabilitation for the Aged

Masayoshi Itoh
Mathew H. M. Lee

Improvements in medical and surgical technology and public health have dramatically increased life expectancy. In 1900 only 4 percent of the United States population was age 65 or over, but by 1980 this had increased to 11 percent. It is projected that by 2030 over 50 million people or 17 percent of the total United States population will be in this age group.[1]

The aged are men and women who worked all their lives and sacrificed to maintain our society, to improve our standard of living, and to assure the future of our children. While the elderly in Eastern cultures may enjoy respect for their wisdom and recognition for their contribution to society, the elderly in the United States may be viewed as a population unproductive and crippled, a national burden.

In recent years our youth have been surrounded by subliminal messages suggesting that there is something so wrong or distasteful about aging that it either should not be seen or should be regarded as a joke. Movies present children, teenagers, and young adults in the leading roles, but since John Wayne died we seldom see an elderly "hero" in films. Television has portrayed the elderly as fatuous and insane, while mimicking their physical and functional limitations. Portrayals in neither medium promote appreciation and respect. Advertisements consistently stress youth and the necessity for superficial youthfulness. The clothing, food, and home products industries rarely utilize a middle-aged or elderly model in the promotion of their wares. Acceptable elderly role models are scarce in the media. Euphemisms such as "senior citizen" and "golden ager" are merely compensatory; they do not change the concepts now held by the younger population.

Those who engage in clinical medicine, particularly rehabilitation, are finding an ever-increasing elderly population who become ill and disabled. So-called geriatric rehabilitation is becoming a large part of the daily practice in the field of rehabilitation. If one is to provide meaningful and supportive rehabilitation services to the aged, stereotyped concepts must be abandoned. Every effort must be made to understand value systems, life-styles, and individual problems of the aged.

One of the pitfalls in scientific discussion is the loose use of a term or terms. Rusk's[2] definition of rehabilitation, "the ultimate restoration of a disabled person to his maximum capacity—physical, emotional, and vocational," seems to be comprehensive enough and has been universally accepted. It is interesting, however, to examine this definition. There are two key phrases, "ultimate restoration" and "maximum capacity." If the emphasis is placed on *restoration,* then the goal of rehabilitation is to bring functional capacity to the premorbid level. If the patient was not functioning at maximum capacity premorbidly, then successful rehabilitation services may achieve a goal higher than restoration. Rehabilitation may make an individual as good as before or better than before. If the patient is adult or aged, the former goal may be applicable. If the patient is a child, adolescent, or young adult, the latter may be more appropriate.

In the field of gerontology and geriatrics, the most ill-defined word is "aged" or "elderly." While evaluating a healthy 50-year-old male traumatic above–knee amputee, a very young resident physician from a developing nation stated, "This patient is too old to have an above–knee prosthesis." His statement astonished as well as amused us. Perception of "old" depends upon each individual's cultural and social background. In order to test this theory, the question "What is your definition of an old person?" was asked of laypersons. Many responded, "A person 65 years of age or older." Until recently the mandatory retirement age was 65, and after the 65th birthday one can receive Social Security benefits. Responders based their answers on the Social Security system rather than on any theory of what constitutes "old." One wonders, now that the mandatory retirement age is 70, what the concept of "old person" will become.

From the womb to death in old age, there are certain benchmarks that divide the epochs of the life of a human being (Figure 1-1). Such benchmarks as newborn, infant, child, adolescent cause very little disagreement. The aging process is a continuous and cumulative process taking place in humans from conception to ultimate death. It is generally agreed that the first two decades of human life is the phase of the productive aging process and that the degenerative aging process commences in the third decade of life. While puberty is generally accepted as the division between childhood and adolescence, few if any would agree that the climacterium is the division between middle age and old age. There seems to be no universally accepted benchmarks after adolescence.

There are certain morphologic and histopathologic degenerative changes that alter one's functional status. These are commonly found among those who are advanced in age. These degenerative changes are insidious, progressive, and irreversible and involve multiple organ systems. When many such changes can be detected objectively or subjectively, the individual may be called "aged." If bio-

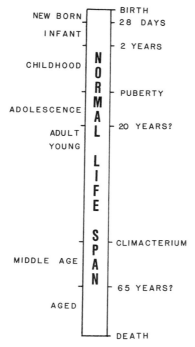

Fig. 1-1.   Benchmarks on a normal life span.

logic or chronologic age is used as a basis for defining "old" or "aged," then it is necessary to make qualifying exceptions and explanations. Many well-known statesmen, scientists, artists, and musicians functioned superbly and were completely capable of pursuing high levels of achievement well into the sixth, seventh, or even eighth decade of life or beyond.

Once in a great while, the description of a patient in the medical record reads, "This is a 70-year-old white male appearing younger than his age," or even "This is a 70-year-young white male." On the other hand, there are many persons in the younger age groups, particularly those who have undergone prolonged physical, emotional, and/or socioeconomic stress, who exhibit very advanced aging processes. However, such deviations are seldom noted in medical records, perhaps because of stereotypic conceptions of aging in the minds of medical and paramedical professionals.

Another aspect of defining the aged is self-conception. Mortimer Collins said, "A man is as old as he's feeling, a woman as old as she looks." John Godfrey Saxe wrote in his *I Am Growing Old:*

> I'm growing fonder of my staff;
> I'm growing dimmer in the eyes;
> I'm growing fainter in my laugh;
> I'm growing deeper in my sighs;

> I'm growing careless of my dress;
> I'm growing frugal of my gold;
> I'm growing wise; I'm growing—yes,—
> I'm growing old!

Rollin John Wells in his poem *Growing Old* stated:

> A little more tired at close of day,
> A little less anxious to have our way;
> A little less ready to scold and blame,
> A little more care of a brother's name;
> And so we are nearing our journey's end,
> When time and eternity meet and blend.

These writings vividly describe persons who recognize the changes of advanced age in their own physical and mental functions and realize they are old. Perhaps the most significant factor that makes a person feel old is the realization that one has some of the characteristics of the aged. Often this comes as a shock even to the older person. The realization may stem from something big or something small. Having to use a cane or wear orthopedic shoes can be just as devastating as recognizing a severe disability. It is vitally important for those who provide care to the elderly to comprehend this psychologically vulnerable state in an individual.

HEALTH STATUS OF THE AGED

Publilius Syrus, now a relatively obscure writer but in his day a popular writer of maxims in the Roman Empire, first century B.C.E., said, "Good health and good sense are two of life's greatest blessings." A Greek poet, Simonides of Ceos, in the sixth century B.C.E. noted in his *Sextus Empiricus:* "There is no joy in beautiful wisdom, unless one have holy health." The Scottish essayist and philosopher Thomas Carlyle stated in 1838: "Ill-health of body or of mind, is defeat. . . . Health alone is victory. Let all men, if they can manage it, contrive to be healthy." Health and ill health have been a great concern of the human race for centuries. Numerous writings related to this subject can be found throughout the literature of many cultures.

The most quoted and widely accepted concept of health is the definition by the World Health Organization (WHO):[3] "A state of complete physical, mental, and social well being and not merely the absence of disease or infirmity." While no one disputes this definition of health, one may wonder if such a condition exists. The existence of a state of complete physical well-being is quite conceivable; the term mental implies in this context not only mental but also emotional and psychological. Today the average intelligent person is concerned about local, national, and international politics, war and peace, future environmental safety, violence and crime, etc. Thus in our contemporary society the state of complete mental well-being may not be achievable. Social well-being includes economic

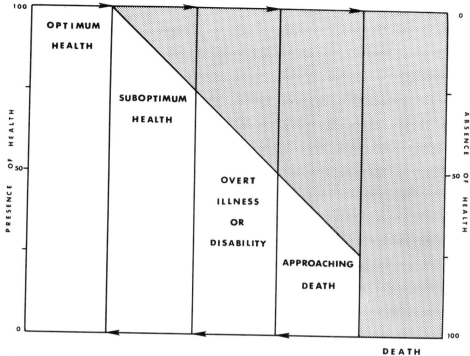

Fig. 1-2. Health status scale. [Modified from E. S. Rogers, Human Ecology and Health, Macmillan Publishing Co., New York, 1960.]

and vocational components. In view of current national and international economic conditions, there are ongoing changes resulting in economic problems and unemployment. Thus presently attainment of perfect health as defined by WHO can be equated to a search for the fountain of youth or immortality.

Therefore it seems to be more appropriate in this chapter to discuss the different aspects of physical health. Rogers[4] developed a conceptual model of human health. This model recognizes five levels or states of health, *Optimum Health* being one extreme and *Death* being the other (Figure 1-2). Assuming the total sum of health to be a constant, Optimum Health represents complete presence of health, and Death represents total absence of health. Optimum Health is the physical health that WHO defined.

However, there is a state that is not Optimum Health but is a state with "absence of disease or infirmity." This particular state is called *Suboptimum Health.* The majority of the aged are in this state of health due to arteriosclerotic, osteoarthritic, or osteoporotic changes that accompany aging, even though they may be asymptomatic.

The state of *Overt Illness or Disability* is usually recognizable. However, illness that has an insidious onset, such as multiple sclerosis or Parkinson disease, may be difficult to detect until the overt symptoms appear.

In spite of the increase in knowledge and understanding of disease processes and the improvement of diagnostic and therapeutic techniques, a disease may progress to a point that threatens life. This state is called *Approaching Death.* Cardiac pacemakers, cardiac bypass surgery, organ transplantation, hemodialysis, etc. may allow those who were in this state of health to return to a relatively normal life in the state of Suboptimum Health. Others in the Approaching Death state can be maintained at this level for weeks, months, or even years if all necessary life-support systems are artificially provided. But these efforts to prolong life or postpone death often become the subject of medicolegal, religious, or ethical controversy. Finally, every man and woman reaches the state of Death. Death by definition is absolute and irreversible. But with effective cardiopulmonary resuscitation, many people previously considered to be dead are returned to the state of Approaching Death.

Once it was thought a human life begins at birth and terminates at death. In recent years there have been fierce debates over the time a human life starts. It is universally agreed that some form of life starts at the time of conception, and two cells, ovum and sperm, eventually become a human being. A dewdrop on a leaf on a high mountain cannot be called an ocean, although this dewdrop may eventually become a part of an ocean. By the same reasoning, not by any stretch of the imagination can these two cells be called a human being. There is life in a cell, life in an embryo, life in a fetus, and life in a human. There seems to be little disagreement in the medical community that a human life starts when the oxygen supply to the body enters through the lungs and ceases to pass through the umbilical cord. The basis of the "when life begins" controversy is perhaps more of an emotional, religious, or legal conflict than a scientific one.

Similarly, there have been disagreements as to the point at which a human being is considered dead. Customarily, death is pronounced when all vital functions cease or no vital signs can be detected. However, with the development of artificial life-support systems, we are able to artificially maintain cardiopulmonary functions, nutritional requirements, and electrolyte and fluid balance. In order to refine the definition of death, the concept of brain death was introduced. If the electroencephalogram, which is a record of brain activity, shows a flat line, brain death is pronounced, even though the electrocardiogram can register cardiac activity because of the use of life-support equipment. In many states, after confirmation of brain death by two physicians and if family consents it is legal to remove body organs for organ transplantation. On the other hand, under the same circumstances, if medical practitioners turn off the artificial life-support systems, they may face criminal prosecution. One thus recognizes that there is no longer one simple definition of death in contemporary medical practice. There is great need for a reappraisal of the definition of death, but one can assume that as science discovers additional means to nullify death other disagreements or problems will arise.

In the Rogers' Health Status model,[4] no human condition remains static at any level of health for a prolonged period. It constantly changes in either direction, down to Approaching Death or up to Optimum Health. The changes of the health status toward Death is a natural process similar to the skier being pulled down the mountain slope by gravity. On the other hand, raising of the health status toward Optimum Health may require a conscious effort. The extent of that effort depends upon the person's health classification. If a human is in Suboptimum Health, simple rest may suffice, but for one in the state of Approaching Death rigorous and sometimes heroic medical and/or surgical intervention may be required, similar to the skier at the bottom of the mountain who uses a ski lift to return to the peak, representative of Optimum Health.

The Rogers' Health Status Scale was devised to apply to the general population and not to a particular subgroup of the population, such as the aged. However, the Rogers model, demonstrating fluidity in human health status, is applicable to the aged. As has been stated, degenerative aging processes begin in the third decade of human life. These processes are natural, inevitable, progressive, cumulative, and irreversible. Such cumulative effects may become clinically more evident in the sixth decade of life. Obviously these aging degenerative changes do not affect all organ systems equally. Such changes may be discovered as incidental findings in a clinical investigation of a totally unrelated physical problem. Nevertheless, it is reasonable to assume that the health status of those who reach the sixth and subsequent decades of life are at best in Suboptimum Health. Currently, medical science has no known method to restore the aged to the level of Optimum Health. Thus the scope of the health status for the aged is more limited and narrower than that of the younger population.

SUSCEPTIBILITY OF THE AGED

In the early twentieth century, Stallybrass[5] defined epidemiology as "the science which considers infectious diseases—their course, propagation, and prevention." Welch[6] defined epidemiology as "a study of the natural history of disease," and Lilienfeld[7] described it as "the distribution of a disease or condition in a population and of the factors that influence this distribution." Sartwell and Last[8] defined it simply as "the study of the distribution and dynamics of disease in populations."

As the evolution of definitions of epidemiology indicates, the focus of this branch of medicine now encompasses communicable diseases and all types of diseases as well as physical and mental disabilities.[9] Clinical medicine, and geriatrics in particular, has dealt with each disease entity of the aged from etiology to treatment. Epidemiologic investigations into the problems of the aged also probe to find the developmental processes of a specific condition, disease, or disability. This is the first step toward a scientific approach to limitation and prevention. Such epidemiologic investigation and analyses employ the same conceptual approach and methodology that is always used to study communicable diseases.

The first consideration in epidemiology is the host and the host's susceptibility. The word "susceptibility" was derived from the Latin word *suscipere*, meaning to receive or undertake. In general use susceptible means "easily affected emotionally" or "having a sensitive nature or feelings." Dorland's Medical Dictionary defines susceptible as referring to "an individual who is not known to have be-

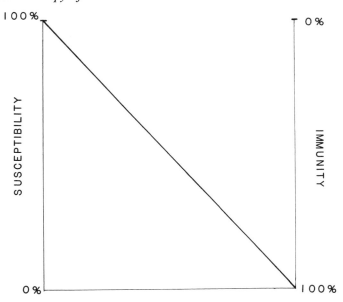

Fig. 1-3.   Relationship between susceptibility and immunity.

come immune to an infectious disease by either natural or artificial means." Immunity is generally regarded as the capacity of an individual, when exposed to infection, to remain free of illness or infection.[8] For example, all human races are susceptible to *Borreliota variolae,* which causes smallpox, unless they have been vaccinated recently. A human who is vaccinated loses susceptibility and gains immunity to variola. Immunity is security against a particular disease or poison. Specifically, it is the power an individual sometimes possesses naturally or acquires to resist and/or overcome an infection to which most people are susceptible.

Susceptibility and immunity are two opposite host reactions to a disease. Immunity and susceptibility, however, may seldom be considered as absolute states. When one is discussing the presence or absence of susceptibility, it is almost the same as discussing the absence or presence of immunity (Figure 1-3).

If a given population is highly susceptible to a disease or condition, that particular group of people is considered to be a high-risk population. It is commonly known that a majority of the aged are least susceptible to the common childhood diseases such as rubella, varicella, or pertussis. This is because most of the aged had these diseases in their childhood and developed active immunity. Statistics show that the aged are less susceptible to highway traffic accidents than adolescents or young adults but more susceptible to automobile accidents as pedestrians. The former is probably due in part to their maturity—they avoid speeding and alcoholic consumption or drug abuse. Thus in this case the aged as drivers are a lower risk population. Pedestrian accidents may be explained by visual and/or auditory disabilities, kinesthetic disturbance, incoordination, slowed reflex time, etc. The visual disability in this case is not hyperopia but possibly a condition such as senile immature cataract. Central or conduction deafness is the common hearing problem of the aged. Kinetic abnormalities, incoordination, and retarded reaction time may be the result of neurovascular degeneration. Aged pedestrians therefore are a high-risk population, since their age-related disabilities make them most susceptible to accidents while walking. It is likely that aged persons subject to these disabilities do little if any driving.

It has been stated that the health status of the aged is at best Suboptimum Health owing to the presence of degenerative aging processes. Each degenerative change may cause a specific disease condition. For example, arteriosclerosis, one of the most common degenerative aging changes, may eventually result in arteriosclerotic heart disease or myocardial infarction. On the other hand, cerebral arteriosclerosis may contribute to the development of Parkinsonism or senile dementia. However, these conditions can hardly be called symptoms of arteriosclerosis, but those who have arteriosclerosis are indeed increasingly susceptible to such diseases.

A multiplicity of degenerative changes associated with aging may increase the susceptibility of the aged to a variety of diseases and conditions. One very common traumatic condition among the aged is fracture of the neck of the femur. There are different theories on whether hip fracture is the result of a fall or the cause of a fall.[10] For this discussion we shall assume that hip fracture is the result of a fall.

Visual disability, kinetic abnormalities, and retarded reaction time have been described previously. Other symptoms, such as syncopic episodes and vertigo, are related to neurovascular degeneration and may also cause a falling accident. Since it is not uncommon for the aged to be taking hypotensive, hypoglycemic, or psychotropic medication, it should be noted that these symptoms may be iatrogenic.

Osteoporosis is another well-known degenerative aging process that makes bones brittle. Bones of children are far more resilient than those of the aged. In a fall children may suffer from green-stick fracture of the forearm. The aged in a similar accident may sustain a Colles' fracture, which has almost become the hallmark of the old. Hip fracture is found most often among aged women, and osteoporotic changes are known to be accelerated by postmenopausal hormone imbalance. Osteoporotic processes are also known to take place when there is a lack or absence of stress to bones in all age groups. Weight bearing and isometric muscle contraction are main sources of such stress. Whatever the rationale may be, the aged tend to lead a sedentary life. This sedentariness, often self-imposed, and lack of physical exercise may also contribute to the progression of osteoporosis.

There are many environmental factors that may be viewed as causative elements for falling accidents. In a given household there may be three generations exposed to the same environment. The grandparents would be less exposed to any hazardous physical conditions in this house, owing to their sedentariness, than the grandchildren, who are physically very active. Nevertheless, the facts show that they (grandmother more than grandfather) are more likely to fall and fracture a hip. This situation indicates that there is also a greater susceptibility to hip fracture among aged females than there is in the younger population.

It is reasonable to assume that the aged are susceptible to certain diseases and conditions and immune to others. This group's specific susceptibility has its origin in degenerative aging changes. While these changes singly can increase susceptibility, in some cases a combination of them may result in a drastic increase in susceptibility. This epidemiologic analysis illustrates the complexity of susceptibility among the aged and is basic to understanding the natural history of disabilities as commonly found in advanced age groups.

DISABILITIES AMONG THE AGED

Edentulous, stooped, with poor vision, hard of hearing, walking with a shuffling gait—a common concept of an old man. Old age is closely associated with disability in the minds of the general public. Various degenerative aging processes can be responsible for the development of disabilities such as hemiplegia, amputation of lower extremities due to vascular insufficiency, hearing loss, senile cataract, organic brain syndrome, or senile dementia. These disabilities are direct results of disease processes and are often called primary disabilities.

In the daily practice of rehabilitation the major effort is not limited to treatment of these primary disabilities but also includes treatment to prevent the development of secondary disabilities. Secondary disability is defined as disability that does not exist at the onset of primary disability but develops subsequently.[9] Examples of secondary disability are flexion contracture of joints, subluxation of the shoulder joint in hemiplegics, decubitus ulcer, and disuse atrophy of muscles. Development of the secondary disability is closely related to a long–lasting primary disability, resulting in spasticity, flaccidity, imbalanced power in antagonists, hypoesthesia or anesthesia of skin, pain, disuse, or immobilization.

The onset of the primary disability is, in general, acute or sudden, while development of secondary disability is often insidious. Flexion contracture of joints in hemiplegics and rheumatoid arthritics may develop over a period of weeks and months. It is not unusual to find an elderly patient with rheumatoid arthritis contracted almost into the fetal position. Such deformities are vivid illustrations of the damage done by long-term illness, pain, lack of proper exercise, neglect, and perhaps by self-resignation.

A decubitus ulcer, on the other hand, may develop in a relatively short period. While contracture of a joint causes kinetic functional deficiencies, a decubitus ulcer could result in life-threatening consequences. An individual with an extensive ulcer loses a large amount of body fluid and consequently dehydration, electrolyte imbalance, and hypoproteinemia ensue. Nutrition for the elderly is often poor. Subcutaneous fat tissues are depleted, and bony prominences protrude directly under the skin. Diminished activity in sebaceous glands makes the skin of the aged less elastic and drier. These common characteristics are the reason that the elderly with primary disability develop an extremely high susceptibility to decubitus ulcer. From the onset the nutritional condition is precarious; appearance of the ulcer upsets nutritional balance further and creates a vicious cycle to the point of cachexia. At this stage there are often multiple decubiti. Another complication of decubitus ulcer is infection, often with gram-negative organisms. Such infection not only destroys surrounding soft tissue but also causes osteomyelitis. Septicemia due to an infected decubitus ulcer is not uncommon.

Certainly in any age group a primary disability may alter one's life-style. The sequelae of secondary disability can put an end to one's life-style and to one's life. Susceptibility to secondary disability in the aged, like primary disability, is a consequence of degenerative aging changes.

Rusk's[2] definition of rehabilitation refers to restoration of the total human being. In order to accomplish this goal, the individual's ability as well as disability must be assessed thoroughly by a group of medical and allied health professionals. Their findings are most often presented in a descriptive and narrative form. To simplify such presentations, methods of rating functional capacity have been devised. Classic examples are the Cardiac Function Classification by the American Heart Association and the Manual Muscle Power Rating by the National Foundation of Infantile Paralysis. These use an ordinal scale with letters or numbers or a combination of the two to indicate the ratings. Whether a letter or number is used, such as F or 3 in muscle power grading, is immaterial as long as each gradation is clearly defined so that the ratings are reproducible. Nominal scales are more descriptive; however, unless the definitions are exceptionally clear they are often confusing. Nominal scales are frequently used when rating Activities of Daily Living (ADL)—e.g., partial independent, minimum assistance, etc.

There are many disability assessment methods, from rather simple ones to lengthy ones that examine not only physical but psychosocial and vocational factors.[11-15] When a numerical scoring system is utilized, certain significant factors are weighted. Workmen's Compensation uses a weighted percentage system, 100 percent being total disability. Most of these methods focus on the general population; there are very few disability rating systems specifically designed for the aged population.

The PULSES Physical Profile by Moskowitz and McCann[16] is perhaps the earliest method in the literature for evaluation of disabilities in the aged. Each of the six letters in PULSES represents a particular category of human function, and each category is rated on a scale of 1 to 4; normal function according to age is indicated by 1 and poorest function by 4 (Table 1-1). Experience in the Skilled Nursing Facility of Goldwater Memorial Hospital over the past 15 years reveals the extremely high reproducibility of PULSES scores. An attending physician in this facility scores a PULSES profile on each admission and annual physical examination. Comparison of two or more PULSES profiles of a patient clearly illustrates progress or regress over the years. Further, individual PULSES records are adaptable to wall charts or card files to provide a comprehensive record of a group's scores. The Moskowitz[16] and the Goldwater groups have independently developed color-coding systems.

Another approach to assessment of disability in elderly people is to measure the amount of assistance required. Long-Term Care Placement Form—Medical Assessment Abstract (DMS-1) by the New York State Department of Health is an example (Figure 1-4). Their form DMS-9 (Figure 1-5) shows the weighted scores of each entry. A total score indicates the amount of nursing care needed. These

Table 1-1. Pulses Patient Profile

P. *Physical condition,* including diseases of the vicera (cardiovascular, pulmonary, gastrointestinal, urologic, and endocrine) and cerebral disorders not enumerated in the lettered categories below.
1. No gross abnormalities considering the age of the individual
2. Minor abnormalities not requiring frequent medical or nursing supervision
3. Moderately severe abnormalities requiring frequent medical or nursing supervision yet still permitting ambulation
4. Severe abnormalities requiring constant medical or nursing supervision confining individual to bed or wheelchair

U. *Upper extremities,* including shoulder girdle and cervical and upper dorsal spine
1. No gross abnormalities considering the age of the individual
2. Minor abnormalities, with fairly good range of motion and function
3. Moderately severe abnormalities but permitting performance of daily needs to a limited extent
4. Severe abnormalities requiring constant nursing care

L. *Lower extremities,* including the pelvis and lower dorsal and lumbosacral spine
1. No gross abnormalities, with fairly good range of motion and function
2. Minor abnormalities, with fairly good range of motion and function
3. Moderately severe abnormalities permitting limited ambulation
4. Severe abnormalities confining the individual to bed or wheelchair

S. *Sensory components* relating to speech, vision, and hearing
1. No gross abnormalities considering the age of the individual
2. Minor deviations insufficient to cause any appreciable functional impairment
3. Moderate deviations sufficient to cause appreciable functional impairment
4. Severe deviations causing complete loss of hearing, vision, or speech

E. *Excretory function,* i.e., bowel and bladder control
1. Complete control
2. Occasional stress incontinence or nocturia
3. Periodic bowel and bladder incontinence or retention alternating with control
4. Total incontinence, either bowel or bladder

S. *Status*—mental and emotional
1. No deviations considering the age of the individual
2. Minor deviations in mood, temperament, and personality not impairing environmental adjustment
3. Moderately severe variations requiring some supervision
4. Severe variations requiring complete supervision

With permission from Moskowitz E, McCann CB: Classification of disability in chronically ill and aging. J Chron Dis 5:342, 1957.

forms are an administrative tool that determines a patient's eligibility for admission to a long-term care facility and are not designed primarily for disability assessment. However, an experienced reviewer of DMS-1 can visualize the state of the individual's health and nursing needs as well as the extent of disabilities from the total score. The shortcoming of this form lies in its ambiguous terminology, which tends to decrease its reproducibility. Studies show that DMS-1 is a reliable method for its original intended purpose.[17, 18]

It is likely that more disability assessment methods will be devised for the increasing elderly population. While most of the disability evaluation methods, including PULSES, attempt to express physical and mental disability directly, measurement of other parameters such as nursing care needs can also illustrate the scope of physical and mental limitations.

PAIN IN THE AGED

While almost all people are subject to pain, somehow nagging muscle aches and joint pains are often referred to colloquially as being caused by old age. There are no statistical data or research substantiating this belief.

Pain is one of the most difficult pathophysiologic phenomena to define. Pain is human perception or recognition of a noxious stimulus in a part of the body. Crue's definition of pain, "anything the patient said it is,"[19] illustrates the mysterious nature of pain. The mystery is due to our insufficient knowledge and understanding of neurophysiology and neurochemistry. There is disagreement among experts on transmission and perception of noxious stimulus, and various hypotheses have been advanced. Melzak's gate theory[20] is representative of the school of peripheralists. To account for various unexplainable symptoms such as hemiplegic pain or thalamic pain, the school of centralists has advanced a theory of central pain. There is also a difference of opinion as to whether phantom pain should be considered as peripheral or central pain. In addition, the newly discovered brain peptides, such as β-endorphin, and their relation to pain are being studied, but information is still inconclusive.

Pain may be classified as acute, chronic, or malignant. Acute pain is characterized as severe, its onset often sudden, with corresponding objective symptoms; owing to the existence of definitive treatment methods, it has a predictable duration and good prognosis. Pain due to trauma such as fracture, laceration, sprain, or acute abdominal infection is an example of acute pain.

Chronic pain may vary from mild to severe. It may follow acute pain, it may begin suddenly or gradually, and it often is recurrent. Corresponding objective symptoms may or may not be present. There is often no effective treatment method, its duration is unpredictable, and its prognosis is guarded. While acute pain is generally considered peripheral pain, some hold that chronic pain may be central pain.[21]

Malignant pain has many of the characteristics of acute pain, but it lacks definitive treatment methods and its prognosis is extremely poor. Malignant pain is

NEW YORK STATE DEPARTMENT OF HEALTH
LONG TERM CARE PLACEMENT FORM
MEDICAL ASSESSMENT ABSTRACT
PREDICTOR SCORE

CURRENT PAT. LOCATION
☐ HOSP. ☐ DCF
☐ SNF ☐ HOME CARE
☐ HRF ☐ OTHER
SPECIFY

REASON FOR PREPARING FORM
☐ DISCHARGE/TRANSFER TO
☐ ADMISSION FROM
☐ REVIEW FOR PERIOD FROM ______ TO
☐ MEDICAID REVIEW ☐ DEATH
☐ OTHER, SPECIFY

PATIENT NAME LAST FIRST M.I. | STREET CITY STATE ZIP | SEX ☐ MALE ☐ FEMALE

PATIENT NUMBERS
S.S. NO.
MEDICARE NO.
MEDICAID NO.
SOC. SERVICE DIST.
MEDICAL RECORD NO.
ROOM NO.

PATIENT DATES
DATE OF BIRTH ______ AGE
DATE LATEST HOSP. STAY -
FROM
TO
DATE THIS ADMISSION
RESPONSIBLE PHYSICIAN

PROVIDER INFO
NAME
ADDRESS
MEDICAID NO.
MEDICARE NO.
DOES PATIENT HAVE PRIVATE INSURANCE?
☐ NO ☐ YES

MEDICAL COVERAGE: PATIENT'S CONDITION AND TREATMENT REQUIRING SKILLED SUPERVISION (ALL ITEMS MUST BE COMPLETED)

1. A. DIAGNOSES OCCASIONING CURRENT USE OF SERVICES:
PRIMARY
OTHER
OTHER
OTHER
B. NATURE OF SURGERY ______ DATE
C. IF PATIENT HAD CVA/MI SPECIFY ______ DATE
D. ALLERGIES OR SENSITIVITIES, SPECIFY

2. LIST SIGNIFICANT MEDS/INJECTIONS.
(FOR PARENTERAL MEDS ALSO CHECK ITEM 3A)
MED DOSE FREQUENCY ROUTE

3. A. NURSING CARE & THERAPY (SPECIFY DETAILS IN 3D, 3E OR ATTACHMENT)	FREQUENCY			SELF CARE		CAN BE TRAINED	
	NONE	DAY SHIFT	NIGHT/EVE SHIFT	YES	NO	YES	NO
PARENTERAL MEDS							
INHALATION TREATMENT							
OXYGEN							
SUCTIONING							
ASEPTIC DRESSING							
LESION IRRIGATION							
CATH/TUBE IRRIGATION							
OSTOMY CARE							
PARENTERAL FLUIDS							
TUBE FEEDINGS							
BOWEL/BLADDER REHAB.							
BEDSORE TREATMENT							
OTHER (DESCRIBE)							

B. INCONTINENT
URINE OFTEN* ☐ SELDOM** ☐ NEVER ☐ FOLEY ☐
STOOL OFTEN* ☐ SELDOM** ☐ NEVER ☐

C. DOES PATIENT NEED SPECIAL DIET? NO ☐ YES ☐
IF YES, DESCRIBE

*MORE THAN ONCE A WEEK **ONCE A WEEK OR LESS

3. D. Is the patient's condition unstable so that an R.N. must detect/evaluate need for modifications of treatment/care on a daily basis?
NO ☐ YES ☐
If yes, describe instability and specific need for nursing supervision, vital signs ranges, lab values, symptoms, etc.

E. Is there high probability that complications would arise in caring for the patient without skilled nursing supervision of the treatment program on a daily basis?
NO ☐ YES ☐
If yes, describe (a) patient's condition requiring skilled nursing supervision (b) the aggregate of services to be planned and managed in the treatment program. Indicate services needed and potential dangers of complicating clinical factors.

F. Circle the minimum number of days/week of complex skilled nursing supervision:
REQUIRES 0 1 2 3 4 5 6 7
RECEIVES 0 1 2 3 4 5 6 7

DMS—1 (1/77)

Fig. 1-4. New York State Department of Health, Long-Term Care Placement Form. Medical Assessment Abstract (DMS-1).

PATIENT NAME	LAST		FIRST	M.I.	PATIENT S.S. NO.	MEDICAL RECORD NO.	ROOM NO.

4. FUNCTION STATUS

FUNCTION STATUS	SELF CARE	SOME HELP	TOTAL HELP	CAN NOT	REHAB* Poten.
WALKS WITH OR W/O AIDS					
TRANSFERRING					
WHEELING					
EATING/FEEDING					
TOILETING					
BATHING					
DRESSING					

5. MENTAL STATUS

MENTAL STATUS	NEVER	SOME-TIMES	ALWAYS		REHAB* Poten.
ALERT					
IMPAIRED JUDGMENT					
AGITATED (NIGHTTIME)					
HALLUCINATES					
SEVERE DEPRESSION * *					
ASSAULTIVE					
ABUSIVE					
RESTRAINT ORDER					
REGRESSIVE BEHAVIOR					
WANDERS					
OTHER (SPECIFY)					

6. IMPAIRMENTS

IMPAIRMENTS	NONE	PARTIAL	TOTAL		REHAB* Poten.
SIGHT					
HEARING					
SPEECH					
COMMUNICATIONS					
OTHER (CONTRACTURES, ETC.)					
SPECIFY					

7. SHORT TERM REHAB. THERAPY PLAN
(TO BE COMPLETED BY THERAPIST)

A. DESCRIBE CONDITION (NOT DX) NEEDING INTERVENTION | SHORT TERM PLAN OF TREATMENT AND EVALUATION & PROGRESS IN LAST 2 WEEKS | ACHIEVEMENT DATE

B. CIRCLE MINIMUM NUMBER OF DAYS/WEEK OF SKILLED THERAPY FROM EACH OF THE FOLLOWING:

REQUIRES / RECEIVES

	REQUIRES		RECEIVES
PT	0 1 2 3 4 5 6 7		0 1 2 3 4 5 6 7
OT	0 1 2 3 4 5 6 7		0 1 2 3 4 5 6 7
SPEECH	0 1 2 3 4 5 6 7		0 1 2 3 4 5 6 7

8. DO THE WRITTEN ORDERS OF THE ATTENDING PHYSICIAN AND PLAN OF CARE DOCUMENT THAT THE ABOVE NURSING AND THERAPY ARE NECESSARY?   NO ☐ YES ☐

9. A. SHOULD THE PATIENT BE CONSIDERED FOR ANOTHER LEVEL OF CARE: NO ☐ YES ☐   IF YES: WHEN? _____   WHAT LEVEL? _____

B. AS A PRACTICAL MATTER, COULD PATIENT BE CARED FOR AS AN OUTPATIENT?   NO ☐ YES ☐

C. AS A PRACTICAL MATTER, COULD PATIENT BE CARED FOR UNDER HOME CARE?   NO ☐ YES ☐
IF YES TO ANY OF ABOVE, ATTACH A DISCHARGE PLAN.

10. SHOULD THE PATIENT/RESIDENT BE MEDICALLY QUALIFIED FOR SNF CARE?   COVERED ☐ QUESTIONABLE ☐ NON-COVERED *** ☐

11. ADDITIONAL COMMENTS ON PATIENT CARE PLAN/REHAB. POTENTIAL _____

12. I CERTIFY, TO THE BEST OF MY INFORMATION AND BELIEF, THAT THE INFORMATION ON THIS FORM IS A TRUE ABSTRACT OF THE PATIENT'S CONDITION AND MEDICAL RECORD.

_____ (SIGNATURE OF DESIGNATED RN AND TITLE) _____   DATE ASSESS. COMPLETED

TO BE COMPLETED BY U.R. AGENT OR REPRESENTATIVE UPON CONTINUED STAY REVIEW

13. ADDITIONAL INFORMATION BY U.R. REPRESENTATIVE

15. U.R. REPRESENTATIVE PLACEMENT _____
SIGNATURE _____ DATE _____

16. U.R. PHYSICIAN: PLACEMENT _____

14. NEXT SCHEDULED REVIEW DATE _____
SIGNATURE _____ DATE _____

*CHECK THE BOX CORRESPONDING TO APPROPRIATE CRITERION IF THERE IS A LIKELIHOOD THAT THE PATIENT WILL RESPOND UNDER A COORDINATED PLAN OF RESTORATIVE TREATMENT. (INDICATE PLAN IN ITEM 3 E OR 11).

**IF PATIENT HAS SEVERE DEPRESSION, PSYCHIATRIC CONSULTATION SHOULD BE OBTAINED.

*** IF CHECKED "NON-COVERED", SNF PLACEMENT CANNOT BE APPROVED BY MEDICAID.

A. ITEMS 1, 2, 3, 4, 5, 6 SHOULD BE COMPLETED BY NURSE
B. ITEM 7 SHOULD BE COMPLETED BY THERAPIST.
C. ITEMS 8, 9, 10, 11, 12 TO BE COMPLETED IN CONSULTATION WITH THE HEALTH TEAM.

DMS-1 (1/77)

New York State Health Department Numerical Standards Master Sheet
Numerical Standards for Application for the Long Term Care Placement Form
Medical Assessment Abstract
(DMS-1)

3.a. Nursing Care and Therapy (Specify details in 3d,3e or attachment)

	None	Frequency Day Shft	Frequency Night/Eve.	Self Care Yes	Self Care No	Can Be Trained Yes	Can Be Trained No
Parenteral Meds	0	25	60	-15		0	0
Inhalation Treatment	0	38	37	-20		0	0
Oxygen	0	49	49	-4		0	0
Suctioning	0	50	50	-1		0	0
Aseptic Dressing	0	42	48	0		0+1	0
Lesion Irrigation	0	49	49	-20		0	0
Cath/Tube Irrigation	0	35	60	-1		0*4	0
Ostomy Care							
Parenteral Fluids	0	50	50				
Tube Feedings	0	50	50				
Bowel/Bladder Rehab.	0	48	48				
Bedsore Treatment	0	50	50				
Other (Describe)	0	0	0				

b. Incontinent

Urine: Often* ☐ 20   Seldom** ☐ 15   Never ☐ 10
Foley ☐ 15

Stool: Often* ☐ 40   Seldom** ☐ 20   Never ☐ 0

c. Does patient need a special diet?   No ☐   Yes ☐

If yes, describe _____

DMS-9 (2/77)

---

4. FUNCTION STATUS

	Self Care	Some Help	Total Help	Can Not
Walks with or w/o aids	0	35	70	105
Transferring	0	6	12	18
Wheeling	0	1	2	3
Eating/Feeding	0	25	50	
Toileting	0	7	14	
Bathing	0	17	24	
Dressing	0	40	80	

5. MENTAL STATUS

	Never	Sometimes	Always
Alert	40	20	0
Impaired Judgment	0	15	30
Agitated (nighttime)	0	10	20
Hallucinates	0	1	2
Severe depression			*
Assaultive	0	40	80
Abusive	0	25	50
Restraint Order	0	40	80
Regressive Behavior	0	30	60
Wanders			
Other (Specify)			

6. IMPAIRMENTS

	None	Partial	Total
Sight	0	1	2
Hearing	0	1	2
Speech	0	10	20
Communications			
Other (Contractures, etc.)			

7. Short Term Rehab. Therapy Plan (To be completed by therapist)

a. Describe Condition (not Dx) Needing Intervention | Short Term Plan of Treatment & Eval. and progress in last 2 weeks. | Achievement Date

b. Circle Minimum number of days/week of skilled therapy from each of the following:

REQUIRES	RECEIVES	
0 1 2 3 4 5 6 7	0 1 2 3 4 5 6 7	PT
0 1 2 3 4 5 6 7	0 1 2 3 4 5 6 7	OT
0 1 2 3 4 5 6 7	0 1 2 3 4 5 6 7	Speech

+ 37 for skilled rehab/therapy (received & required both > 0)

Fig. 1-5. New York State Health Department Numerical Standard Sheet (DMS-9).

caused by malignant tumors in their terminal stage. Obviously this classification is based on methods of clinical management rather than any other consideration.

It seems more reasonable to group pain into two categories, acute and chronic. Chronic pain may be subgrouped into an acute-chronic model and a recurrent-chronic model (Figures 1-6, 1-7, and 1-8). In the acute-chronic model the precise point when pain changes clinically from acute to chronic is unknown.[22]

Treatment of the etiology is the choice for management of acute pain. A liberal use of narcotic analgesics to free the patient from discomfort is the acceptable approach to malignant pain, and in such cases the possibility of addiction should not prevent the use of narcotics.

On the other hand, *the chronic pain which is frequently observed in the aged is most difficult to control* and is a challenging task for clinicians. Chronic pain, particularly the recurrent type, may or may not be accompanied by objective findings. Even if such findings can be treated surgically, such as a herniated disk, there is no guarantee that pain will be totally eliminated after the surgery. Pain is a somatic and subjective symptom, and chronic pain may not always correspond to any objective findings. The degree and extent of pathologic or abnormal findings are not necessarily indicators of severity and chronicity in pain.

It has been well recognized that emotional and socioeconomic factors play an important role in the causation of chronic pain. While tension and anxiety are normal emotional reactions to the presence of severe acute pain, various complex psychologic factors may contribute to chronic pain. Chronic situational depression is often due to a realization of aging, loneliness, or unmet socioeconomic needs; it is frequently found to be the contributing emotional factor.

As with other somatic complaints, careful evaluation of the physical condition is the best basis for developing a management plan for chronic pain. Even if a definite pathology, such as osteoarthritic change, is found, the investigation for the source of chronic pain should include the psychosocial state of the patient. Such comprehensive assessment is fundamental to establishing a rational and meaningful patient care plan.

The constant presence of pain, even intermittent nagging pain, interferes with normal activities of daily living. Self-imposed immobilization will result in joint contractures, causing severe disability. A feeling of isolation and the development of deformities would aggravate a precarious emotional balance. Therefore every effort should be made to eliminate the pain or to make it more tolerable.

In the management of chronic pain a surgical approach is usually not the first choice of treatment. Various nonnarcotic analgesics can be prescribed, but the aged are more susceptible to the cumulative effects as well as side effects. Some patients may be under a medication regimen for an illness totally unrelated to the condition causing the pain. In such cases possible drug interaction between other medications and analgesics must be carefully considered. When a psychologic state such as chronic situational depression is an outstanding component of chronic pain, antidepressants may be prescribed. There are also a variety of physical therapy modalities that are effective to lessen discomfort. In addition, it is important to remember that psychologic and social counseling are also helpful.

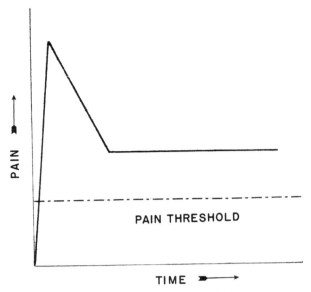

Fig. 1-6.   Acute pain model.

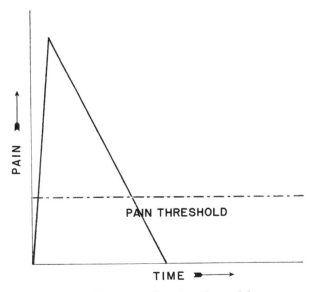

Fig. 1-7.   Acute–chronic pain model.

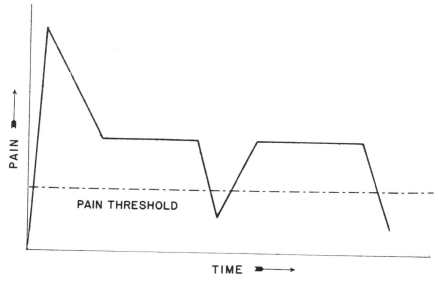

Fig. 1-8.   Recurrent chronic pain model.

GERIATRIC REHABILITATION

Advancement in medical knowledge and technology since the turn of the century is unprecedented in human history. While the first half of the twentieth century is marked by great contributions to the understanding of diseases, the latter half of this century has been a period of superspecialization in the field of clinical medicine. For the past two decades the terms *geriatric rehabilitation* and *pediatric rehabilitation* have been used. Does this mean the users of these terms advocate a subspecialty in rehabilitation medicine? Probably not. It is more than likely done to emphasize certain characteristic approaches to rehabilitative care specially designed for the two age groups. In this chapter the term geriatric rehabilitation is used to signify certain other conceptual and practicable aspects of rehabilitation for the aged.

As mentioned previously, the goal of rehabilitation for the aged is restoration of physical function to the premorbid level. The aged population's high susceptibility to certain primary and secondary disabilities and a health status that is at best suboptimum have also been discussed. The images of the aged drawn from these discussions indicate the distinctly different characteristics of their disabilities and rehabilitation.

Prior to development of the treatment strategy, an assessment of the premorbid life-style, functional level, and health status is mandatory in geriatric rehabilitation. In general, the younger population maintains a certain life-style according to occupations and social obligation. They maintain Optimum Health most of the time and are able to perform not only all activities of daily living (ADL) but can participate in rigorous recreational activities as well.

On the other hand, it is difficult to generalize about the aged population. One person may follow a very sedentary life pattern, while another may enjoy a life-style as active as someone decades younger. Some may be assisted by relatives and friends in ADL, while many others are functioning physically and mentally at their optimum level. Although it is true that various degenerative aging processes are present, not every elderly person is ill and infirm. In these respects more exceptions will be found among the aged than among the younger population.

The primary goal of geriatric rehabilitation is so limited that the health care team must have a clear understanding of the *functional level to be achieved through the rehabilitation process.*

A careful assessment will provide a clearer picture of the patient and indicate what may be achieved by the individual. This will help the patient establish realistic goals. In addition, a thorough evaluation of the physical condition is mandatory prior to initiation of physical restoration because such evaluation will reveal the extent of the aging processes. This evaluation includes not only routine physical examination but cardiopulmonary functions, peripheral blood circulation, degree of osteoporosis if so indicated, as well as mental condition. Findings from these assessments would suggest the patient's endurance, indications or contraindications for certain treatment regimens, the pace of the rehabilitation process, and possibly prognosis of final functional ability.

After the acute onset of the primary disability, a patient often requires relatively protracted bed rest until he or she is ready for rehabilitation. Such prolonged inactivity will decondition anyone, including young people. The degree of deconditioning is more severe in elderly people, even if they led active lives premorbidly. Thus regardless of disability the most important step in beginning a rehabilitation process is general conditioning to build up endurance. If this conditioning process is omitted, cardiovascular or respiratory disturbance may ensue. Once such complications develop, not only will the rehabilitation process be interrupted and delayed but the patient may become fearful of the process and withdraw into depression. This physical conditioning period is also an excellent time to prepare the patient for resuming as normal a life as is possible in the future.

Sometimes the process of geriatric rehabilitation can be agonizingly slow. The reasons for this slow progression are many; some are psychological, and others are physical. Shyness, resentment, shame, anger, and depression interfere with the performance of even simple physical exercise. Members of the rehabilitation team must be able to appreciate these feelings and play supportive roles. Physically, elderly persons may have neuromuscular incoordination, delayed reaction time, and diminished vision and hearing. Their muscle power may not be strong enough to perform a demanded task. Physically elderly persons may have good days and bad days. One day they may be very energetic and perform extremely well; on another day they may not be able physically to muster the required energy to perform the same task. This does not indicate regression. Elderly people merely lack the "reserves" of youth and can no longer "push" themselves to function beyond a certain point. Furthermore, they may have difficulty remembering and may simply forget what was taught the day before.

The key word for therapists is "patience," and they must be able to understand these subtle mental and physical characteristics of the disabled aged. Words of empathetic encouragement by a therapist are more effective than scolding. Repetition of the same physical action, though necessary, can be dull and boring. The patient may begin to feel that repetition is necessary due to some deficiency within himself or herself. The therapist must interpret the reasons for repetitive exercise, and sincere praise by the therapist, even for slight progress, can promote self-confidence, fortitude, and motivation. Self-confidence is believing that a task can be done; fortitude is the strength, courage, and endurance to do it; and motivation is the desire to do it.

The fear of falling is another very common phenomenon among the aged. Sometimes this fear is so strong that a patient is petrified and refuses to get out of a wheelchair. An analysis of this fear indicates that the source of fear is the fall itself rather than the consequences, such as fractures. This fear is particularly common among women who did not participate in some sort of sport when younger. One approach for this type of patient is to provide maximum physical support, such as direct physical contact or contact guarding by a therapist while a second therapist stands next to the patient. The patient is more confident knowing that two therapists will be able to prevent a fall. Once sufficient confidence is established, these supportive measures may be gradually withdrawn.

Another, more complex method is to condition the patient. This has been done with actors and athletes for many years. In involves training the patient to fall without injury by practice-falling onto a mattress. However, the patient must be constantly supervised and the therapist must be specifically trained in falling techniques in order to teach them.

Regardless of patient age, every opportunity should be given the patient to gain maximum restoration of function. For example, it is often said that a patient "is too old to use an above–knee prosthesis." Age per se is not a contraindication. There must be some irrefutable reason, such as cardiac or respiratory deficiency, extreme weakness, flexion contractures in the lower extremities, poor muscle coordination, or lack of trainability due to poor memory, to deny the patient a prosthesis. It is both a fallacy and a misconception to believe that rehabilitation potential is equated with patient age.

PREVENTIVE REHABILITATION

Efforts to restore health from Overt Illness or Approaching Death to Optimum Health are usually called therapeutic medicine. In a broad sense the goal of therapeutic medicine is restoration of health to the premorbid level. Considering the definition of rehabilitation, one might call therapeutic medicine an "act of rehabilitation."[23] As previously discussed, rehabilitation for children and adolescents may restore physical, intellectual, and/or vocational function to a state better than the premorbid level, but this exception cannot be applied to therapeutic medicine.

The restorative and curative aspects of clinical medicine can be illustrated in acute and episodic illnesses such as acute appendicitis, upper respiratory infection, or acute gastroenteritis. However, when clinical medicine is applied to a chronic disease, these same aspects become less distinct. For example, a given patient with arteriosclerotic heart disease goes into acute cardiac decompensation. Control of acute congestive heart failure usually is not very difficult, and within a few days cardiac function would be restored. This patient will most likely be on a maintenance dose of a cardiac medication for a long period. At this point therapeutic medicine becomes preventive medicine because administration of a maintenance medication prevents a recurrence of congestive heart failure. Here it is easy to see how the distinction between therapeutic and preventive medicine becomes less prominent. A similar meld exists for therapeutic rehabilitation and preventive rehabilitation.

A cursory observation of the activity of physical therapists, occupational therapists, and nurses gives the impression that they are engaged in restoration of disabilities. However, a close analysis reveals that a major part of their effort is to prevent secondary disabilities such as joint contractures, disuse atrophy, osteoporosis, or decubitus ulcer. If these preventive activities were not mandatory, the rehabilitation process would be much simpler and faster. To stress this aspect of rehabilitation the term *preventive rehabilitation* was introduced.[23–25]

Contemporary therapeutic rehabilitation concentrates on the treatment of primary disability and the prevention or treatment of secondary disability. Once primary disability develops in a person, rehabilitation processes cannot always achieve a complete restoration. Even if full restoration is accomplished, it costs the patient as well as the community time, energy, resources, and emotional anguish. Preventive rehabilitation focuses on prevention or eradication of both primary and secondary disabilities (Table 1-2). Some may argue that this is preventive medicine and should not be a part of rehabilitation, which is a therapeutic specialty; however, it should be noted that today there are many components of preventive medicine in every clinical specialty.

The aged population is susceptible to various disabling diseases and conditions. Residual disabilities often interfere with their normal daily functions, and they may need assistance at home or care in an institution. Thus preventive rehabilitation is most meaningful for this population.

Various public health measures, discoveries, and innovations in preventive medicine are practiced in the United States and worldwide in order to prevent numerous infectious diseases and decrease potentially disabling diseases and conditions. Some of these preventive measures are more effective than others. For example, a well-planned and properly executed vaccination program can eliminate poliomyelitis in a given geographic area; on the other hand, well-publicized high-

Table 1-2. Components of Rehabilitation

Disability	Rehabilitation	
	Therapeutic	Preventive
Primary	Treatment	Prevention Eradication
Secondary	Prevention Treatment	Prevention Eradication

school driver education programs have not had the expected impact on highway fatalities.[26] A major focus of preventive medicine has been the population of childhood, adolescence, young adult, and middle-age adult. It appears that the aged are somewhat neglected in this area.

Certain preventive rehabilitation measures for the aged should start before a person has become "aged," e.g., in their 30s and 40s. Hypertension is one of the most common causes of cerebrovascular accident; however, in recent decades the incidence of cerebrovascular accident due to hypertension has drastically decreased because of advancement in drug therapy and other means of controlling hypertension. Early detection and proper control of diabetes mellitus may prevent diabetic retinopathy, peripheral neuropathy, or peripheral vascular insufficiency. If these are combined with meticulous foot care, lower extremity amputation due to diabetic gangrene may be prevented in the advanced age group. Physicians who treat patients with these diseases should stress both the importance of controlling these diseases and the preventive aspects of the treatment regimen. Unless patients and their families understand both therapeutic and preventive aspects of the prescribed treatment, they may not adhere to the regimen as strictly as they should.

In considering other aspects of preventive rehabilitation for the aged it is necessary to assess susceptibility to certain diseases or trauma. For example, fracture of the neck of the femur is found almost exclusively in the aged population, particularly in females. The physical characteristics of this population cannot be altered. Therefore the preventive measures must be environmental. Neatness in the home, improved lighting, and handrails on steps and stairways are examples of environmental protection. An elderly woman with shuffling gait should be encouraged to wear shoes instead of house slippers, and throw rugs should never be used in a household where elderly persons live.

Primary health care personnel who treat the aged, such as physicians, hospital nurses, visiting nurses, physical therapists, or occupational therapists, must recognize the danger of falling accidents among the elderly. Dizziness or transient cerebral ischemic attack is one of the most common causes of a fall, aside from environmental obstacles. Some such attacks are drug-induced, while others may be due to vascular spasm. Therefore health care personnel should give instructions to the aged and those who help them as to what they should do in case of a dizzy spell.

Hip fracture is a common injury among hemiplegics who have successfully completed rehabilitation. The fracture occurs almost invariably on the side of paralysis, probably because of muscle weakness. As part of a prosthesis-rehabilitation program a lower extremity amputee is routinely trained in the technique of falling. If all hemiplegics are trained how to fall by a physical therapist during their rehabilitation, the incidence of hip fracture among hemiplegics may decrease.

The above examples of preventive rehabilitation illustrate that some measures are designed primarily for prevention of primary disability and that others are indirectly preventive. Many existing means of preventive rehabilitation and the need for new approaches and preventions can be identified by continued analysis of the susceptibility of the aged to primary disability, medical care practices, and community action and services on behalf of the elderly. Levy and Moskowitz[27] state, "A focus on prevention means educating the public and health professionals alike on how to obtain information on risk factors or ways to change life-styles and habits or means to promote behavioral changes."

The concept of preventive rehabilitation is rational, and obviously its potentials are unlimited. The question is, *Who*, logically, should be responsible for this health problem of the elderly? The members of the rehabilitation team have a wealth of knowledge on the natural history and treatment of primary and secondary disabilities. The team practices comprehensive care for the total human being. Its practice is not confined to physical therapy, occupational therapy, hospital patient room, private office, or clinic, but includes years of consistent action at the community, state, and federal levels. This concerted effort has in the past resulted in many changes that have improved the quality of life for those who are handicapped and those who are not. Those who engage in rehabilitation are the best equipped to undertake this new frontier of geriatric rehabilitation.

REFERENCES

1. Butler RN: Introduction. In: Second Conference on the Epidemiology of Aging, eds. Haynes SG, Feinleib M. Washington D.C., U.S. Dept. of Health and Human Services, NIH Publication No. 80-968, 1980.
2. Rusk HA, Hilleboe HE: Rehabilitation. In: Preventive Medicine, eds. Hilleboe HE, Larimore GW. Saunders, Philadelphia, Pa., 1965.
3. World Health Organization: Constitution of the World Health Organization. Geneva, World Health Organization, 1964.
4. Rogers ES: Human Ecology and Health. Introduction for Administrators. Macmillan, New York, 1960.
5. Smillie WG: Preventive Medicine and Public Health. Macmillan, New York, 1952, chap. 18.
6. Welch WH: Institute of Hygiene. In: Rockefeller Foundation Annual Report. New York, 1916.
7. Lilienfeld BE: Epidemiologic methods and inferences. In: Preventive Medicine, eds. Hilleboe HE, Larimore GW. Saunders, Philadelphia, Pa., 1965.
8. Sartwell PE, Last JM: Epidemiology. In: Public Health and Preventive Medicine, ed. Last JM. Appleton-Century-Crofts, New York, 1980.
9. Itoh M, Lee M: The epidemiology of disability. In: Handbook of Physical Medicine and Rehabilitation, eds. Krusen FH, Kottke FJ, Ellwood PM. Saunders, Philadelphia, Pa., 1971.
10. Itoh M, Dasco MM: Rehabilitation of patients with hip fracture. A clinical study of 126 cases. Postgrad Med 28:134, 1960.
11. Knapp ME: Disability evaluation, 1. Postgrad Med 46:184, 1969.
12. Knapp ME: Disability evaluation, 2. Postgrad Med 46:201, 1969.
13. World Health Organization: Classification of disability resulting from leprosy, for use in control program. Bull WHO 40:609, 1969.
14. Sokolow J, Silson J, Taylor EJ, Anderson ET, Rusk HA: A method for the functional evaluation of disability. Arch Phys Med Rehabil 40:421, 1959.

15. Pool DA, Brown RA: A functional rating scale for research in physical therapy. Texas Rep Biol Med 26:133, 1968.
16. Moskowitz E, McCann CB: Classification of disability in chronically ill and aging. J Chronic Dis 5:342, 1957.
17. Foley WJ, Schneider DP: A comparison of the level of care predictions of six long-term care patient assessment systems. Am J Public Health 70:1152, 1980.
18. Harris JF, Orr M, Allaway NC: Long-term care criteria and standards agreement with professional placement determination. Am J Public Health 72:602, 1982.
19. Crue BL, Felsoory A, Agnew D, Kaindar MD, Randle W, Griffin S, Sherman R, Menard P, Pinsky JJ: The team concept in the management of pain in patients with cancer. Bull Los Angeles Neurol Soc 44:70, 1979.
20. Melzak R: The gate-control theory of pain. In: The Puzzle of Pain, ed. Melzak R. Basic Books, 1973.
21. Crue BL: A physiological view of the psychology of pain. Bull Los Angeles Neurol Soc 44:1, 1979.
22. Itoh M, Lee MH: Epidemiology of pain. Bull Los Angeles Neurol Soc 44:14, 1979.
23. Itoh M, Lee M: The future role of rehabilitation in community health. Med Clin North Am 53:719, 1969.
24. Itoh M: Preventive rehabilitation for leprosy—A new approach to an old problem. Rehabil Rev 19:13, 1968.
25. Karat S: Preventive rehabilitation in leprosy. Leprosy Rev 39:39, 1968.
26. Robertson LS, Zador PL: Driver education and fatal crash involvement of teenaged drivers. Am J Public Health 68:959, 1978.
27. Levy RI, Moskowitz J: Cardiovascular research: Decades of progress, a decade of promise. Science 217:121, 1982.

2 | Biological Aspects of Aging

Barrie Pickles

This chapter summarizes the major biologic changes that occur during normal aging in those tissues of the body of particular significance to the physical therapist. The effect of these aging changes on function are outlined, and suggestions for dealing with these clinically relevant changes are put forward.

GENERAL PHYSIOLOGIC PRINCIPLES

Claude Bernard pointed out many years ago that all physiologic mechanisms are designed to facilitate one goal—that of maintaining constant the composition of the internal environment of the body. Two basic principles are involved in all physiologic control mechanisms: (1) the Arndt-Schultz principle and (2) the law of initial values.

Arndt-Schultz Principle

This principle is as follows (Figure 2-1):

1. The application of a subthreshold level of stimulation produces no change in the physiologic system.
2. The application of a suprathreshold level of stimulation will result in an increase in physiologic function.
3. The application of a supramaximal level of stimulation will reduce the level of function and may cause destructive changes to occur.

Although this general principle applies to persons of all ages, it has special clinical implications for elderly clients. First, a greater amount of stimulation is

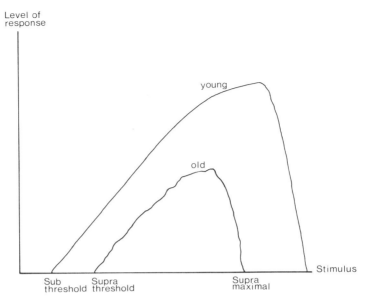

Fig. 2-1. Level of response, young versus old persons.

required for an aging patient before any physiologic response is obtained. This means that if the therapist uses the same level of stimulation (e.g., heat, cold, vibration, traction) and is conservative in approach, it is possible to undertreat the elderly patient. The result is the (mis)interpretation of the lack of response to mean that there is no response to be obtained from the patient and that true rehabilitation potential will never be achieved. Second, the level and type of response resulting from the application of a given stimulus is usually lower and less predictable for the aged than for younger clients.

Finally, elderly patients experience the peak level (supramaximal) of therapeutic response sooner than the young. The practical implication is that the total range of safe therapeutic intervention is smaller in the elderly than in the young.

Law of Initial Values

With a given intensity of stimulation, the degree of change produced tends to be greater when the initial level of that variable is low—the higher the initial value, the smaller the change produced.

If the composition of the internal environment (the homeostatic level) is maintained at a completely steady level, the application of a given stimulus would always produce a similar degree of response. In life, the homeostatic level fluctuates up and down over time. Some physiologic functions vary in a regular, cyclic fashion; these are referred to as biorhythms. Those whose cycle is 24 hours are termed diurnal variations. In normal young adults the sequence of many different biorhythms is highly coordinated.

In older individuals the biorhythm cycles become less regular, and greater variations occur between the high and low values of a particular variable than occur in younger subjects. As the result of increasingly irregular fluctuations in the level of physiologic activities in older persons, the amount of response following the application of a particular stimulus becomes more variable and less predictable.

Clinically, the law of initial values has grave implications for the organization of rehabilitation care of the aged. First, evaluation of a patient's current ability and capacity for improvement must not be based on only one evaluation. What is the time of day that this patient is most alert and able to participate? Scheduling of evaluations as well as therapeutic intervention should be customized to the biorhythms of each individual patient as much as possible. The reality is that it may mean that the physical therapy staff may need one staff member to work from 7 AM to 3 PM and another to work from 11 AM to 7 PM to be able to facilitate the patient's ability to learn by providing treatment during his or her time of greatest physiologic efficiency each day. The whole structure of rehabilitation care will need to be examined to assure that it supports the stabilization of biorhythms of each individual patient.

Other patterns of activity that need to be customized to each patient include wake/sleep patterns, eating, and activity cycles. This customized scheduling is difficult in an institutional environment and is a strong argument for an increasing emphasis on home-based rehabilitation for the aged when feasible. The goal of this attention to detail is to avoid any unnecessary disruption of biorhythms that already (due to normal aging) tend to be increasingly uncoordinated.

FIBROUS CONNECTIVE TISSUE

All connective tissue cells have a common ancestry—all develop from the same primitive type of mesenchymal cell. As the result of this common ancestry connective tissue cells have many features in common, with special stress being placed on one particular function. All connective tissue cells secrete collagen, elastin, glycoproteins, hyaluronic acid, and contractile proteins. In different tissues the proportion of each of these substances varies; in white fibrous tissue the predominant secretion is that of collagen, in yellow elastic tissue elastin is particularly prevalent, and in cartilage the glycoprotein secretion is especially common. Under different environmental conditions within the body, the pattern of secretions by connective tissue cells will be altered. The production and functional significance of each of these secretions is summarized below, and the effects of aging on each are considered.

Collagen

Ribosomes of connective tissue cells produce a secretion of procollagen, a protein material.[1] Molecules of procollagen are then extruded from the cell into the surrounding tissue fluids. Once they have left the cell the individual procollagen molecules stick together end-to-end to form a strand of tropocollagen. Later a number of tropocollagen strands come together as the result of electrical attraction between the strands; one part of each strand is positively charged, while other sections of each strand are negatively charged. Later, chemical bonds also develop between adjacent tropocollagen strands, causing the strands to become tightly wound in a spiral fashion to form a mature collagen fiber.[2,3]

Tropocollagen is quite soluble in cold water; as the conversion of tropocollagen into collagen occurs, and as maturation of the collagen fibers progresses, the fiber becomes progressively more insoluble. The greater the number and type of chemical bonds that have developed between the strands, the more insoluble the material becomes. Newly developed collagen is still soluble in dilute acid, but fully mature collagen is quite insoluble.

Collagen fibrils grow in diameter by the surface aggregation of additional tropocollagen strands. As this occurs the collagen in the center of the fiber is compressed and becomes more dense. The growing fiber is characterized by a central portion of intermolecularly cross-linked insoluble collagen surrounded by less completely cross-linked material.[4]

The eventual diameter of the fibers depends on the chemical composition of the matrix in which they are embedded. Even when the fibers have reached their ultimate size, further cross-linkages continue to be added. At this stage the nature of these later cross-linkages is chemically different from those developed in the earlier stages.[5]

The diameter of collagen fibers in a given location in the body is usually greater in old persons than in younger subjects. The increased diameter of these fibers is possibly a reflection of the chemical changes in the matrix in older persons and the addition of more tropocollagen to the surface of the collagen fiber. When the oxygen concentration in the matrix is moderately low, the secretion and maturation of collagen continues to take place, even when other secretions have ceased. In general therefore the tensile strength of connective tissue in older persons is greater than that of younger adults.

In two situations, however, there will be a reduction in the tensile strength. The initial secretion of procollagen by the fibroblasts is hampered in patients suffering from scurvy. Vitamin C is required to convert the amino acid proline into hydroxyproline, a component of the procollagen molecule.[6] Many elderly persons suffer from a vitamin C deficiency. Chronic stress, also a problem for a large number of old people, has an inhibitory effect on collagen secretion and maturation.[7]

Elastin

Elastin is also secreted by ribosomes within the connective tissue cells of children and younger adults. When elastin molecules are brought together in the extracellular fluids the molecules link up with each other not only end-to-end but also in a branching arrangement, thus creating a lattice-type network of elastin material. As its name implies, elastin possesses the power to recoil to its original length after it has been stretched and the stretching force has been removed.

The amount of elastin in the skin, the bronchial tree, and in the walls of larger arteries is reduced progressively during life.[8] If overstretching of part of an elastin network occurs in adults and elastin fibers are torn, healing by scar tissue will follow. The elastic properties of these tissues (skin, the bronchial tree, arterial walls) will therefore be progressively reduced during life.

Glycoproteins

Glycoproteins are substances formed when polysaccharide carbohydrate material links with protein molecules. The presence of glycoproteins in the extracellular area produces an osmotic force that is important in maintaining the fluid content of the tissues. The glycoproteins (or mucopolysaccharides) form a group of relatively small molecules of soluble protein material. The higher the concentration of glycoprotein molecules in the extracellular fluids, the greater will be the amount of fluid retained within the tissue by osmotic attraction forces. The production and liberation of these glycoprotein molecules by the connective tissue cells is considerably reduced in old age; thus it becomes progressively more difficult for the tissues to retain their normal fluid content, and so progressive dehydration will occur in the tissues of elderly people.

A number of different glycoprotein secretions have been identified. The mixture of glycoproteins varies among different tissues and may alter in a particular location as part of the aging process.[9] There appears to be a definite relationship between the type of glycoprotein present and the thickness of collagen fibers found in different tissues. In the elderly, for example, where dermatan sulfate is the predominant glycoprotein in the skin, the collagen fibers that are formed have a greater average diameter than those in younger subjects, in whose tissues chondroitin sulfate is the most predominant glycoprotein. In the skin of elderly persons, the increased average diameter of the collagen fibers may be largely accounted for by an increase in the dermatan sulfate secretion; the corresponding dehydration of the skin would indicate that although the secretion of dermatan sulfate had increased, the total glycoprotein secretion was reduced.

The function of collagen production and glycoprotein production are independent of each other. Strains of fibroblasts have been grown that produce only glycoprotein, but no cells have been found that secrete only collagen.

Hyaluronic Acid

Some ribosomes in the connective tissue cells produce hyaluronic acid, which helps to regulate the viscosity of the tissues. Friction between different cellular components during movement or as the result of biochemical activity will be reduced to a minimum if adequate amounts of hyaluronic acid are produced. In older persons the secretion of hyaluronic acid by the connective tissue cells is reduced; the viscosity of the connective tissues is altered, and movements tend to be more difficult or are prevented.

Contractile Proteins

Contractile proteins are secreted to some degree by all types of connective tissue cells. The presence of contractile proteins in these cells gives them the power of motility—the ability to push out a pseudopodium to ingest a particle of tissue debris, the power of some cells to move bodily within the tissue spaces, the capacity to force a way through the wall of a capillary or lymphatic vessel. The presence of contractile proteins within a cell is by no means restricted to muscle fibers; indeed, muscle fibers betray their mesenchymal origin by the presence of contractile proteins within their substance. The reduced motility of connective tissue cells in older persons may be explained in terms of reduced secretion and organization of the contractile proteins within these cells.

Some Clinical Problems of Aging in Fibrous Connective Tissue

Fibrinous Adhesions. During life a small but regular exudation of molecules of the soluble plasma protein fibrinogen occurs through the capillary wall into the neighboring tissue spaces, where they will be converted into sticky strands of insoluble fibrin. These adhere to nearby structures in a random fashion and tend to restrict movement of these structures. These fibrinous strands will be broken down during the performance of normal activities, and the debris is removed by scavenging reticuloendothelial cells.

In the elderly the exudation of fibrinogen into the tissue spaces is increased; more fibrin tends to be deposited in the tissue spaces of older persons than in those of younger individuals. If activity is not maintained, complete breakdown of fibrin may not occur. Increased amounts of sticky fibrin may accumulate in the tissue spaces and produce adhesions, which will restrict movement between adjacent structures. Fibrinous adhesions also form in a localized area following damage to the tissues.

In many cases restoration of regular normal activity is sufficient to cause breakdown of fibrinous adhesions, but in some cases, when the mass has become consolidated, it may be necessary for stretching to be applied using passive movements or even manipulation under anesthesia.

Collagenous Contractures. As secondary chemical bonds develop between adjacent collagen strands during the maturation process to bring the tropocollagen fibrils more closely together, other bonds are produced that cause shortening and distortion of the collagen fibers. Shortening of the collagen fibers through this mechanism may result in the production of contractures. As more collagen fibers in a mass of connective tissue are shortened in this way, a progressive restriction of movement may be observed.

Collagen fibers are tough and inelastic, and the linking chemical bonds are too strong to be broken down by mechanical stretching forces. Some of these bonds, however, are temperature-sensitive. At 42.5 ° C and above these bonds become unstable and may then be broken. It has been shown that in order to stretch contracted collagen fibers three conditions have to be met:

1. The collagen must be heated to 42.5 ° C or above;
2. A continuous stretching force must be applied while the tissues are being heated;
3. The stretching force must be maintained for at least the first 30 minutes of the cooling period.[10]

Ultrasound may be used to raise the temperature of the collagen to the required level, using a continuous beam with a frequency of 1 MHz at an intensity of 1.0 watts/cm^2 for a period of 10 minutes.

In practice, any soft tissue contracture should be regarded as a mixture of fibrinous adhesions and collagenous shortening. In newly developed contractures the proportion of the total problem attributable to the presence of fibrinous adhesions is high, whereas in more chronic contractures collagenous shortening will predominate. If attempts at normal activity are insisted upon, some improvement in the degree of contracture will result from a breakdown of the fibrin strands. When collagenous shortening is present or interlinking chemical bonds have been established between adjacent collagenous structures, only breaking down these bonds through the use of heat, or correction of the deformity by surgery, will lead to improvement.

Myofibroblast Production. In normal fibroblasts the secretion of contractile protein is only small. Under certain conditions, as the result of a combination of stimuli that are not completely understood, the production of actin and myosin may be increased to a significant extent. Connective tissue cells that produce unusually large amounts of contractile protein are termed myofibroblasts.[11]

The response of connective tissue cells to damage or irritation normally occurs in two stages. In the first stage some cell multiplication occurs, which is followed by a second phase during which the newly increased number of cells become actively secretory. If considerable hyperplasia has occurred before the secretory phase is begun, and if the production of actomyosin is unusually large, the contractile force exerted by the developing mass may be sufficient to prevent normal range of movements in the affected area.

In some older persons this process occurs in the fibroblasts of the rotator cuff at the shoulder to give rise to a particular form of frozen shoulder, in which restriction of movement becomes progressively worse during a 6-month period, remains at its severest level for the next 6 months regardless of the treatment given, and takes a further 6 months to clear. Myofibroblasts are also found in Dupuytren's contracture.

Cartilage

Cartilage tissue is formed when primitive mesenchymal cells are subjected to compression forces in an environment of low oxygen concentration. Under these conditions the predominant secretions of the chondroblast will be a glycoprotein—chondroitin sulfate—and hyaluronic acid, with collagen also being produced to a lesser degree.

Cartilage differs from other tissues in that it has no direct blood supply. Nutrients are supplied to the chondroblasts from blood flowing in the adjacent bones and from the synovial fluid in the joint cavity. The glycoprotein secretions from the chondroblasts pass from the cells into the surrounding matrix where these molecules exert a strong osmotic force to attract water with dissolved gases, inorganic salts, and organic materials into the matrix. In this way materials necessary for normal metabolism are made available to the cartilage cells. The amount of fluid drawn into the cartilage depends on the concentration of glycoproteins in the matrix. During normal aging the production of chondroitin sulfate is reduced[12] and the osmotic attraction forces are lessened, and thus the ability of the matrix to attract and retain fluid is impaired.

The entry of materials into the cartilage matrix is possible only when no compression forces are being applied to the cartilage. When compression is applied, water and dissolved substances are squeezed out. In order to provide for regular movement of materials into and out of the cartilage compression needs to be alternately applied and released. In the absence of compression metabolites remain in the matrix and the oxygen content will be lowered. In response the chondroblast will reduce its secretion of glycoproteins and increase the amount of procollagen produced. Lack of normal activity results in the conversion of hyaline cartilage to fibrocartilage.

Hyaline cartilage covers the articular surfaces in synovial joints. Lubrication between two surfaces of hyaline cartilage is facilitated by the secretion of hyaluronic acid by the chondroblasts. A layer of hyaluronic acid molecules forms a viscous covering on the surface of the hyaline cartilage with a reserve store of these molecules being retained in the cartilage matrix. When compression is applied, more of these molecules are squeezed onto the surface of the articular cartilage. The trapping of synovial fluid in the gaps between these molecules ensures that lubrication of the joint is maintained during movements.[13]

Secretion of hyaluronic acid is decreased during aging, thus reducing the effectiveness of lubrication in the joints of elderly persons. The degenerative changes of aging in cartilage are not reversible. Attention can only be directed toward reducing the possibility of further degenerative changes by subjecting the cartilage to regular but not excessive compression and relaxation forces. This is best achieved by ensuring that older persons maintain their normal activities, particularly those of a weight-bearing type.

Commentary

With normal aging there are notable changes in the activities of all connective tissue cells. It is also common to note that the level of physical activity (cardiovascular as well as general flexibility) decreases with advancing age. The normal age-related changes in connective tissue cells tend to promote less movement or to restrict the ease of movement:

1. Collagen tensile strength is increased.
2. Elastin production is not present with advanced age, and the elastic properties of the tissues (i.e., skin, bronchial tree, arterial walls) is progressively reduced.
3. Glycoprotein production and liberation is reduced, resulting in progressive dehydration of tissues.
4. Hyaluronic acid is secreted less in older persons, resulting in decreased viscosity of the connective tissues.

5. A reduction in secretion and effective organization of contractile proteins make removal of tissue debris less effective.

The combination of a decreased activity level in older persons with the normal age-related changes in connective tissue lead to an impact on the person's ease of desired movement and slowly promote a deterioration of functional capacity. *The key to preventing the normal age-related changes from affecting functional capacity for ease of movement during the entire lifespan is a gradually increasing adherence to a program of physical fitness.* As the person ages, physical fitness becomes more and more important in order to compensate for the normal age-related changes in connective tissue. Prevention of dysfunction due to lack of physical activity must be an emphasis for healthy senior citizens as well as a principle of rehabilitation management of the older patient.

BONE AND THE AGING PROCESS

Normal Bone Development

All types of connective tissue develop from a common type of mesenchymal cell. If primitive mesenchymal cells are subjected to mechanical tension in conditions of low oxygen concentration they become fibroblasts, whereas the application of compression under similar conditions of low oxygen concentration will result in their transformation into chondroblasts. When compression occurs in the presence of higher concentrations of oxygen the primitive mesenchymal cells become osteoblasts.

The development of bone takes place in two stages.

Stage 1. In the first stage the organic component of the bone is laid down. The undifferentiated mesenchymal cells migrate ahead of the capillaries; the leading cells therefore exist in conditions of low oxygen concentration. The application of tension to the cell at this time results in the production of procollagen by the ribosomes within the cell. Once liberated from the cell the procollagen will first be converted into tropocollagen and then into collagen fibers. These collagen fibers will be laid down predominantly along the lines of mechanical stress to become the organic matrix of the developing bone. Within a given plate (lamella) of bone the collagen fibers pass in a single direction; lamellae on either side of this will have their collagen fibers passing in a different direction. The secretion of procollagen is facilitated by the presence of vitamin C.

When compression forces are applied to this area while the blood supply remains poor and the oxygen concentration remains low, the mesenchymal cells respond by producing chondroitin sulfate. This substance passes into the surrounding area to fill the spaces between the collagen fibers that have been laid down. A progressive hardening of this cartilaginous matrix will occur, although inorganic salts and small protein molecules may readily permeate this matrix.

Stage 2. The second stage of bone development results from the improved oxygen content in the region once the capillary network catches up with the migratory mesenchymal cells. After the collagen has been laid down approximately 8 to 10 days pass before this second stage commences. As the oxygen concentration in the area increases, parts of the active mesenchymal cells tend to break away from the general mass of the cell bodies. These cellular fragments, with many enzyme-containing mitochondria, pass into the intercellular matrix.

The most significant enzyme for bone development contained in these fragments is alkaline phosphatase. The presence of alkaline phosphatase in the matrix causes inorganic calcium and phosphate ions to react together to form crystals of hydroxyapatite, or bone crystals. Initially, the hydroxyapatite crystal is attracted to a particular point on the collagen fiber by electrostatic forces created piezoelectrically. The piezoelectric charges are developed as the result of intermittent compression of the developing tissue. Growth of these bone crystals within the matrix continues until all the spaces between the collagen fibers have been filled, providing that the oxygen concentration in the area remains high and intermittent compression of the area is continued. The availability of calcium salts in the developing bone mass is increased through the action of vitamin D.

The deposition of calcium and phosphate ions in the developing bone is regulated through hormonal control. Calcitonin produced by the thyroid gland encourages the deposition of calcium salts in the matrix and their development into bone crystals; the secretion of parathormone by the parathyroid glands tends to have the opposite effect. The balance of activity between these two hormones controls the degree of calcification of the matrix.

Bone is a very active tissue; a constant exchange occurs in both the organic and inorganic components of the bone. Bone is therefore subject to a constant remodeling process, which continues throughout life in response to changes in the functional forces to which the bone is subjected, changes in the availability of calcium and phosphate ions, and shifts in the hormonal balance.

AGING CHANGES IN BONE

The bones of older persons invariably are less dense than bones in younger subjects. The reduction in density may be the result of a failure in the development of both the organic and inorganic components of bone, a condition known as osteopenia, or through defective or abnormal mineralization of the matrix—osteomalacia. The term osteoporosis tends to be applied to any condition where reduction in bone density has occurred, without distinguishing which component is deficient.

SENILE OSTEOPOROSIS

Cellular Changes. Senile osteoporosis would appear to be an extension of the developmental process rather than a degenerative disease of old age.[14] The normal reduction in bone density found in older subjects whose general activities have been progressively restricted may be compounded by a wide variety of pathologic problems.

Pathologic osteoporosis has been related to diets chronically deficient in calcium[15] and to those high in dietary acid derived from meat and poultry.[16] Osteoporosis follows neoplastic infiltration of bone[17] and increased secretion of parathormone[18] and ACTH.[19]

During aging osteocytes undergo degenerative changes—reduction in RNA production, protein synthesis, and mitochondrial activity. The functional activity of the cells is reduced, and glycogen, lysosomes, and age pigment accumulate in the cell bodies.[20] Aging does not alter the ability of skeletal cells to respond to trauma; the degree of response is reduced, however.

Cells responsible for bone resorption and removal are known as osteoclasts. These are large, multinucleated cells having large numbers of mitochondria and acid phosphatase, which are formed by fusion of cells in the osteogenic layer.[21] Osteoclastic activity does not appear to be greatly affected during aging. The progressive loss of bone that occurs during aging results from an increasing difficulty in replacing bone that has been lost.

The timing of changes with age differs in periosteal and endosteal cells. Endosteal bone cells show consistently higher biochemical activities than periosteal cells of similar type, and age changes appear much later at the endosteum than they do at the periosteum.[22]

Bone mineral content starts to decline at about age 40 to 50 years, with a subsequent loss of 10 percent per decade.[23] The rate of bone mineral loss is directly related to the amount of mineral present at maturity; i.e., subjects with higher mineral content lose bone at rates equal to average or faster, and those with lower mineral content lose bone at rates equal to average or slower. In men the mean rate of loss of bone during aging is linear. In women the rate of bone loss in the early postmenopausal period is significantly faster than in older women, suggesting that it follows an exponential rather than a linear pattern.

However, if the rates of bone loss in older adults are compared, the loss in both sexes follows a linear pattern. At this stage the percentage rate of bone loss in females is less than that of males of the same age, reflecting the lower bone density of females at maturity. It is possible that apart from bone loss associated with hormonal changes at the menopause, the lower amount of bone in the elderly of both sexes could be primarily attributed to age-associated decreased activity of daily living.[24]

Decreased activity, leading to a reduction in the normal stresses and strains placed on the bone, is a major factor in the development of osteoporosis in the elderly. During the first stage of bone development a reduction of stresses and strains on the tissues will result in lowered production of procollagen and chondroitin sulfate; if these intermittent forces are reduced in the second stage, attachment of bone crystals to the collagen fibers will be hampered.

Weight Bearing and Muscle Action. Two mechanisms, weight bearing and muscle action, have been described as being important in maintenance of the normal density of the bones.

When the effects of bed rest on normal subjects were investigated, it was found that a decrease in bone mass was detected within 2 weeks; the calcium lost from the bones was excreted in the urine. This loss of calcium occurred in all bed-ridden subjects, whether normal or sick, male or female, young or old. The nitrogen output did not show any consistent response. Exercise on a bicycle ergometer by the patient in the supine or sitting positions failed to change the course of the calcium excretion. Supine exercise up to 4 hours per day did not decrease the urinary calcium output previously elevated by complete bed rest. Quiet sitting for 8 hours combined with 16 hours of lying did not prevent the rise in calcium output. On the other hand, 3 hours per day of quiet standing proved to be sufficient to induce a slow decline of the elevated calcium excretion in four out of five subjects. When the subjects resumed their normal up-and-about activities, both the nitrogen and calcium excretion rapidly decreased below the baseline value of the individual.[25]

Weight bearing alone, although helpful, is not necessarily adequate. Patients with poliomyelitis affecting muscles of the calf, who were involved in a program of standing on the affected limbs for up to 3 or 4 hours a day failed to demonstrate any increased density in the bones of the calf and foot.[26]

Activity alone, without weight-bearing compression, appears to be equally ineffective in preventing or reducing decalcification. Rapid decalcification occurred in the bones of astronauts during weightless space flights even though a stringent program of exercise was performed during the flight.

It would appear that simultaneous compression of the bone and activity of the overlying muscles is necessary to produce electrical potentials within the bone sufficiently high to stimulate bone growth. The piezoelectric effect results from fluctuations in the hydraulic pressure exerted by the bone marrow during weight-bearing activities.

Intramedullary pressures remain steady during slow loading of the bone. During rapid dynamic loading, however, a slight rise in intramedullary pressure is observed. Contraction of the overlying muscles produces an even greater increase in the intramedullary pressure. The initial rise in marrow pressure resulting from fast loading and muscle contraction is followed by a slow reduction; a return to the baseline level is found when the load is removed, but the level remained elevated above the resting baseline level in the muscle contraction experiments until the muscle fully relaxed.[27]

The greatest rise in intramedullary pressure is found when loading of the bone and contraction of the overlying muscles occur simultaneously.

When slow loading is applied the blood can easily escape through the venous channels without causing the intramedullary pressure to rise. With faster loading the intramedullary pressure will be increased until an appropriate volume of blood has been ejected from the marrow cavity. Contraction of the overlying muscles compresses the venules emerging from the bone. The increased intramedullary pressure will be maintained until the muscles relax and allow the trapped blood to escape; the stronger the muscle contraction, the greater will be the rise in intramedullary pressure.

It seems likely that the variations in bone marrow pressure during everyday activities, particularly when these are of a weight-bearing character, create the piezoelectric influences that regulate the remodeling and reconstruction processes of bone tissue.

Management of Patients with Senile Osteoporosis. Osteoporosis is an almost inevitable accompaniment of old age in both men and women. It would appear advisable, then, to regard osteoporosis as a normal feature of the aging process. If this concept is accepted the approach to the management of osteoporosis in the elderly should be directed toward ensuring that bone physiology continues as normally as possible as a person grows older. Basically this amounts to ensuring that regular, adequate, and sufficient production of piezoelectric stimulation to the bone matrix continues. This may be achieved by the application of mechanical strains (compression, tension, and torsion) to the bone while the overlying muscles are in a state of contraction.

Bassett[28] has described a program of exercises for bedridden patients in which axial compression is applied intermittently to the bones of the lower limb by means of a sling passing under the arch of the foot. Bassett's program requires the patient to pull on this sling four times a minute for 15 minutes, four times a day. At first loading is applied gradually and is less than 10 lb; after the first week gradual loading is replaced by rapid loading and the pull is progressively increased to 50–100 lb, depending on the patient. This program has been used successfully in a variety of clinical situations to produce increased density and cortical thickening of bones in the lower limb.[28]

It would appear desirable to supplement Bassett's regimen with exercises for muscles of the lower limb while the compression loading is applied. Bassett shows the sling passing under the foot immediately under the ankle joint to obtain maximum axial compression. From Kumar's data[27] it may be inferred that alternate contraction of the plantar- and dorsiflexors of the ankle with successive compression loadings would produce a greater rise in intramedullary pressure and piezoelectric signal generation than would occur from compression alone. Once the patient can satisfactorily perform this alternate dorsi- and plantar-flexion movement (an isotonic contraction), the exercise may progress so that a simultaneous cocontraction of both dorsi- and plantar-flexor muscles (an isometric contraction) is produced as compression is applied.

Progression should also be made to the performance of these exercises with increasing weight bearing. For patients who have been confined to bed for extensive periods of time the modified compression loading/exercise programs may be practiced on the tilt table, gradually increasing the vertical angle of the table until the upright position and full normal weight bearing is possible.

It should be remembered that Bassett was dealing largely with bedridden orthopedic patients; for ambulatory patients the early stages of Bassett's approach are clearly inappropriate. If a patient is already weight bearing or independently mobile, it will obviously be of little benefit to apply a few pounds of axial compression force through spring-resisted axial-loading exercises performed in the lying position. At the start of the program the therapist must ensure that the total loading applied to the bones is greater than would occur during the patient's normal activities; otherwise no therapeutic benefit can be expected.

What emerges from this line of thought is that elderly persons should engage in weight-bearing activities and exercises not only to retain or improve their cardiovascular fitness or increase their muscle strength but also to prevent or reduce osteoporosis and to facilitate ongoing remodeling and reconstruction of bone.

Most geriatric patients, as well as elderly nursing home residents, participate in group exercise and activity programs. These activity sessions should include as much weight-bearing activity as possible if the best effects on bone are to be produced. Exercises that alter the amount of weight on each foot, attempts to balance on one foot, raising the heels off the floor, arm-swinging exercises from the standing position, ball-catching activities, and passing articles between standing group members all involve shifts of motion, changes in the forces applied to the lower limb, and alterations in the patterns of activity in the muscles that ensheathe the weight-bearing bones. All these activities will develop changing piezoelectric potentials and stimulate normal bone physiology.

Fractures in the Elderly

As progressive structural weakening occurs in bones during aging the likelihood of fractures increases. Bone loss is most evident from the trabecular patterns in the endosteal areas of the vertebral bodies and in the long bones. In the vertebral bodies, which have a particularly high proportion of endosteal bone, osteoporosis tends to occur earlier and be more pronounced than in other bones. Thus the frequency of fractures of the vertebral bodies of older persons is particularly high.

An inverse relationship has been claimed between the degree of osteoporosis and the incidence of fractures in the vertebral bodies and the femoral neck,[29] but this simple relationship has been challenged.[30] Although the mean levels of bone density in both males and females who have suffered fractures of the femoral neck are lower than for the general population in each age group, considerable variance in bone density was found. These results fail to support the hypothesis that there is a single critical level of bone mass below which a fracture of the bone is likely to occur. Other factors appear to be involved.

Lumbar vertebral bodies fail during in vitro experiments when pressures lower than those experienced during normal in vivo situations are applied.[31] During life bones may be considerably strengthened hydraulically by the intramedullary fluid pressure.[32] When compression forces are applied to a bone either through weight bearing or as the result of voluntary muscle action the venules emerging from the bone will be occluded by the action of the overlying contracting muscles, and the outflow of blood from the marrow cavity will be reduced or prevented. The hydraulic pressure within the bone marrow will be raised as a result. The hydraulic support provided by the bone marrow through this mechanism reduces the stress that would otherwise have been placed on the bone trabeculae.[27]

In the elderly not only is the bone less dense than in younger subjects, but the reflex reaction time for muscle contraction during falls is prolonged and the force of the muscle contraction is reduced. Therefore the hydraulic support mechanism to the bone is less effective in the elderly than in younger subjects, thus increasing the risk of damage to the bones of elderly persons from the application of a given force.

The likelihood of stress fractures occurring in osteoporotic bone will be reduced if the overlying muscles are able to contract forcefully and fast. The generalized osteoporosis of senescence is, perhaps, an indication that, in the past, forces applied to the bone have been inadequate to produce full replenishment of bone during the ongoing remodeling process. If exercises to strengthen weakened muscles and increasingly fast rhythmic stabilization exercises to improve their speed of isometric response and fixator capacity are administered, improvement will be noted in the muscle action well in advance of any increase in bone density.

Osteomalacia

Osteomalacia results from a lack of vitamin D. Humans can synthesize vitamin D in the presence of sunlight but also may supplement diet to provide adequate intake. Osteomalacia is found less frequently in people living in areas with long hours of sunshine. In a city in Northern England, where the total number of hours of sunshine each year is low, a high incidence of osteomalacia has been noted.[33] Lower incidence is likely in most parts of the United States because of adequate sunshine and vitamin D supplementation of food.[24]

As it is not possible to distinguish by x-ray examination among senile osteoporosis, pathologic osteopenia, and osteomalacia, vitamin D is often given to all patients with reduced bone density, although its use will lead to improvement only in cases of osteomalacia.

Commentary

With normal aging a decrease in the density of bone has been observed. The mechanisms of healthy bone remodeling are dependent on two variables that can be used as clinical tools: compression of the bone intermittently and the activity of the overlying muscles. All rehabilitation strategies for the aged should incorporate these concepts and avoid the misconceptions that exercise in the supine position will work to prevent bone demineralization. To prevent the unnecessary complication of bone demineralization due to bed rest and sitting in chairs, programs of activity involving intermittent weight shifting/weight bearing should be incorporated into daily care of each aged patient and into preventive programs for the well elderly.

MUSCLE AND THE AGING PROCESS

Normal Muscle Tissue

Skeletal muscle fibers are large, cylindrical multinucleated cells with a diameter between 10 and 100 μ and a length of up to 40 cm. Each fiber is surrounded by a plasma membrane, the sarcolemma. The fiber contains a number of segments, called sarcomeres, arranged end-to-end along the length of the fibers. The sarcomere is the basic contractile unit of the muscle fiber. It contains thick and thin protein filaments of myosin and actin arranged in a regular fashion to produce the characteristic cross-striations of the fiber in an alternate light and dark pattern, enzyme-filled mitochondria, and ribosomes for protein synthesis within a fluid matrix.

Forming a network around the sarcomere is a closed system of tubules, the sarcoplasmic reticulum, in which calcium ions are retained. Nerve impulses cause the liberation of calcium ions from the sarcoplasmic reticulum into the sarcomere, and cross-bridges are established between the myosin and actin filaments. The formation of these cross-bridges causes a sliding movement to occur between the two sets of filaments, with subsequent shortening of the sarcomeres and therefore of the muscle fiber. The calcium ions then return into the sarcoplasmic reticulum, the cross-bridges are broken, and the muscle fiber reverts to its original length.

Energy to produce the movement between the myosin and actin filaments comes largely from the breakdown of adenosine triphosphate (ATP) into adenosine diphosphate (ADP). As only a small amount of ATP is available in the muscle fibers, the ADP will need to be rebuilt into ATP as quickly as possible. Most ATP production takes place in the mitochondria, which are found close to myofibrils where the ATP is required.

Mitochondria in type I fibers contain enzymes that work relatively slowly on free fatty acids under aerobic conditions to produce the energy required to restore ADP to ATP. In type II fibers different enzymes act upon carbohydrate materials under anaerobic conditions to produce this restoration more quickly. Type I fibers are often termed slow fibers and type II fibers fast fibers. Some muscle fibers, termed type IIa fibers, possess both oxidative and glycolytic enzyme systems.

In order to maintain aerobic functioning for as long as possible, aggregations of myoglobin exist in the sarcoplasm of type I fibers. The presence of myoglobin in the fiber facilitates the passage of oxygen into the fiber and also provides for some oxygen storage.

In some animals all the muscle fibers in a particular muscle belly are of the same type, but in humans type I and type II fibers are intermingled in each muscle belly, although the proportion of each type varies from one muscle to another. All muscle fibers in a particular motor unit—i.e., supplied by the same nerve fiber—are of the same type, however.

AGING CHANGES IN MUSCLE TISSUE

The direct effects of age on skeletal muscle are difficult to assess because increasing age and decreasing physical activity are highly correlated. *If skeletal muscles are used frequently, they show remarkably few structural and functional changes with age.* It may be more reasonable to define most of the changes seen in the muscles of elderly persons more as characteristics of disuse rather than of age.

Chemical Changes During Aging

The changes that occur in muscle during aging may involve the following:

1. Loss of fluid and inorganic salts;
2. Changes in enzyme activity;
3. Reduction in contractile proteins;
4. Cellular disintegration.

Loss of Fluid and Inorganic Salts. A rapid loss of fluid from the muscle fibers, together with a loss of dissolved inorganic salts, occurs when injury or disease affects the locomotor system. Within an hour or two following injury to a joint, a reduction in size of the overlying muscles may be noted.

Under normal conditions the sarcolemma acts as a selectively permeable membrane, resulting in an imbalance of potassium and sodium ions on the two sides of the membrane; sodium ions are largely being prevented from entering the muscle fiber, while potassium ions pass readily through the sarcolemma into the muscle fiber and are then retained within the cell. This results in a high intracellular concentration of potassium ions.

A rapid loss of fluid from the muscle fibers occurs when injury or disease affects the locomotor system. This situation is accompanied by a loss of the dissolved inorganic salts, especially potassium ions, from the cell. As the result of degenerative changes to the sarcolemma during aging a slow but progressive loss of fluid and potassium salts occurs from the muscle fiber.[34] It is possible that this problem may be compounded by a lack of potassium ions in the diet. It has been reported that elderly subjects tend to select foods low in potassium.

Lack of potassium ions in the aging muscle reduces the maximum force of contraction that the muscle is capable of generating. The subject complains of tiredness and lethargy. The characteristic variations in these features on a day-to-day basis in an elderly person most likely results from fluctuations in the potassium ion content of the tissues.

The dehydrated elderly patient shows an obvious loss of muscle bulk and is weak and lethargic. Many patients admitted to chronic care institutions in this stage are referred for strengthening exercises and general activities. Little improvement can be expected if the tissue dehydration is not corrected; the greatest improvement is possible only if the proper potassium ion concentration of the tissues is restored. If the blood chemistry is properly attended to by the physician, a dramatic improvement in the physical capabilities of the patient will usually result. Careful monitoring of dehydrated patients receiving potassium ion supplements is necessary to detect any signs of cardiac arrhythmia that may be produced.[35]

In most cases reduction in muscle bulk in elderly patients is due to dehydration and altered ionic concentrations in the tissues rather than resulting from more complex degenerative changes within the muscle.

Changes in Enzyme Activity. Most enzymes in the muscle fiber are contained in the mitochondria. The mitochondria in type I fibers contain oxidative enzymes; in type IIa fibers some mitochondria contain oxidative enzymes and others glycolytic enzymes; and only glycolytic enzymes are present in the mitochondria of type IIb fibers.

Changes begin to occur in muscle enzyme function within 2 or 3 days of cessation of normal activity. These changes first occur—and are most apparent—in the glycolytic enzyme systems of type IIb fibers, although if inactivity persists the oxidative enzyme systems of type I and type IIa fibers may also become involved.[36]

Reduction in enzyme activity will result in a reduced capacity of the muscle to break down food materials to provide energy. This lessening in enzyme activity may be reflected in a reduction of the enzyme content of the mitochondria within the muscle fibers. It is unusual, however, to find a reduction in the number of mitochondria within the muscle fibers resulting from disuse or aging.

Degenerative changes in the mitochondrial enzyme systems are reversible. If activity is commenced or increased, improvements in the enzyme concentration of the muscle mitochondria may begin to appear within a few days, even in the muscles of elderly subjects, although the rate of redevelopment will be slower than in younger persons.[37]

Reduction in Contractile Proteins. Changes to the contractile protein complex in the muscle fibers—true atrophy—only occurs to a limited extent, and then only as the result of prolonged inactivity or degeneration. Some authorities claim that the breakdown of the actomyosin complex will occur only if denervation is present. Others suggest that while degeneration of the contractile elements does not occur before the age of 65, it is possible that after that age some degeneration may take place. In these cases it is suggested that although the nerve cell and axon in a motor unit may remain structurally unaffected, some of the terminal axon filaments may cease to conduct nerve impulses, thus leaving some but not all of the muscle fibers within the motor unit in a denervated condition. In those muscle fibers that have lost their nerve supply, breakdown of the contractile complex will result. The unaffected fibers are required to carry an increased load and may hypertrophy as a result.[38] Examination of a cross-section of such a muscle under the microscope will reveal considerable variation in the diameter of the muscle fibers, whereas in normal muscle the diameters of muscle fibers within a single area of the muscle are remarkably similar. Breakdown of the contractile complex tends to occur first, and is most apparent, toward the outside of the muscle fiber, with the center of the fiber being relatively unaffected.

Neuropathic changes in the muscle appear to be the most common finding in muscles of persons over age 60. The most important factor in the changes of senile muscle is a decrease in the number of functional motor units.[39] These changes have been reported in approximately 30 percent of all persons over age 60, with no increase found in those over age 80. In contrast, the selective atrophy of type II fibers, which occurs in conditions of disuse and malnutrition, increases from 30 percent in the 60- to 70- and the 70- to 80-year-old groups to 50 percent in the 80- to 90-year-old group.[40]

Disintegration of the Muscle Cell. In the event of fluid loss, changes in electrolyte balance, reduction in mitochondria, and breakdown of the contractile complex the muscle fiber reverts to a more primitive form of connective tissue cell. Ribosome function in the degenerate cell shifts from a production of specialized actomyosin to an increase in the degree of procollagen production. Alternatively, if the degenerative changes are sudden or especially severe, breakdown of the nuclei within the muscle fiber may occur or the nuclei may be extruded from the fiber. In either case, death of the fiber will occur, with gradual absorption of the debris by migrating reticuloendothelial cells.

Changes in Neural Activity

Muscle fibers within a motor unit all possess similar characteristics—all are either type I or type II fibers. This finding suggests that the chemical composition of a muscle fiber is dependent on neural control, at least to some degree. Neural control is effected through two mechanisms—(1) by the pattern of nerve impulse activity in the motor endplate area, and (2) by the exudation of neurotrophic substances across the neuromuscular junction, independent of impulse activity.

There is a difference in the frequency of nerve impulse activity to slow and fast muscle. In order to produce a tetanic contraction nerves supplying type I fibers carry impulses at a frequency of 25–30 per second, while 50–60 impulses per second are required to produce a tetanic response in type II fibers. Under laboratory conditions it has been shown that when type I fibers are subjected to chronic stimulation at a high frequency they come to resemble type II fibers more closely, and their contraction time shortens. Conversely, chronic application of slow frequency stimulation to type II fibers will result in a lengthening of their contraction time.[41] Although many questions remain, from these experiments it appears safe to conclude that the normal frequency of impulse activity has some influence on the chemical composition of the muscle fiber. During the normal aging process the patterns of nerve impulse activity do not alter significantly. It appears unlikely that changes in the chemical composition of the muscle fibers result from changes in nerve impulse activity in vivo.

Acetylcholine and other neurotransmitters are liberated in small amounts from the end plate, independent of impulse activity in the nerve. These substances have a trophic, or nutritive, effect upon the muscle fiber. While some of these neurotransmitters may be manufactured and stored in the end-plate region, others are thought to be produced in the body of the nerve cell or in other parts of the neuron, from where they move slowly along the axon to the end plate, and across to the muscle fiber. Some trophic substances move along the axon at speeds as low as 1 mm/day, although others move more quickly. These trophic neurotransmitters are of particular importance in regulating the activity of enzymes for the rebuilding of ATP in the muscle following contraction; if this activity is reduced, contraction times lengthen.

If denervation occurs, both impulse activity and neurotrophic influences on the muscle fiber will be lost. Loss of innervation leads to a dedifferentiation between type I and type II fibers, with each reverting to a more primitive form of cell. In type I fibers the most profound change is in the loss of oxidative enzymes;

in type II fibers an equivalent loss of glycolytic enzymes occurs. The differences between type I and type II fibers are progressively reduced.

There is little or no evidence of degeneration in the end plates as the result of aging, even when extensive changes are found in the muscle fibers. Some reduction may be noted in the number of mitochondria and vesicles present in the end plate, particularly on those that terminate on the surface of type II fibers, but this reduction is not extensive. A reduction in the size and number of junctional folds at these end plates may reduce the capacity for materials to pass across the membrane.

Changes in Blood Flow Through the Muscle

The transfer of metabolites across the capillary membranes within the muscle is reduced in senescent muscle because of increased thickness of the basement membrane of the capillaries, a decrease in the density of the capillary network, and a diminished reaction of blood vessels in senescent muscle to chemical and nervous stimulation.

Degeneration of the basement membrane of cells that form the capillary wall follows the same pattern as that noted previously for muscle and nerve cell membranes. Changes in the surrounding connective tissue add further to the difficulties of transfer of metabolites to and from the muscle fibers.

Three sets of blood vessels, each separately controllable, exist in skeletal muscle bellies. One set of vessels is responsible for the nutrition of the supporting connective tissue, and two sets are responsible for the nutrition of the muscle fibers. The muscle fiber vascular bed consists of two parallel pathways, one of which is influenced by changes in the concentration of hormones in the circulating blood and one which is controlled through autonomic stimulation.[42]

Vasodilation occurring in muscles at or before the commencement of exercise is a response to alterations in the concentration of hormones in the circulating blood, unaccompanied by any change in the metabolic rate of the muscle. During exercise further vascular changes result from changes in the pattern of autonomic nerve activity in the working muscles. In the elderly both these mechanisms become less effective, resulting in a decrease in the degree of circulatory response possible in the working muscles when exercise is performed. It therefore is evident that older persons will be able to perform less work than younger individuals before anaerobic conditions develop in the working muscles.

Commentary

Preventive care is the key to aging changes in muscle tissue. If skeletal muscles are used frequently, they show remarkably few structural changes with advanced age. The majority of changes noted in muscles of elderly persons are characteristics of disuse rather than age. The presumption for effective muscle function is that internal homeostasis exists with adequate hydration and mineral balance. In cases where patients are known to be or are suspected of being dehydrated, with concomitant symptoms of tiredness, lethargy, and general weakness, examination of blood chemistry to assure appropriate balance is a prerequisite to effective physical therapy intervention.

THE NERVOUS SYSTEM AND AGING

Aging is often characterized by reduced sensibility, reduced coordination, reduced cognitive abilities, and a reduced ability to react to changing circumstances. A general assumption is made that loss of nerve tissue is a predominant feature of aging. In reality, although some loss of nerve cells does take place during the aging process, the extent to which this loss occurs is less than usually assumed. The reduced level of nervous system functioning in the elderly is better explained in terms of biochemical changes that take place in neurons during aging and senescence.

Loss of Neurons

The weight of the brain is reduced in old age; there is a 5 percent loss in weight by age 70, 10 percent by age 80, and 20 percent by age 90.[43] It is also accepted that the volume of the brain is reduced to a similar degree.[44]

Reduction in weight and size of the brain has usually been assumed to result from a progressive loss of nerve cells in the brain over a period of time. In an early study it was shown that there is an age-related loss of Purkinje cells from the cerebellar cortex[45] and that a definite loss of neurons from the hippocampus also occurs.[46] In most areas of the brain, however, it has not been possible for age-related neuronal loss to be shown.[47]

From these studies it would appear that although some neuronal loss does occur as part of the normal aging process, this degenerative process does not affect all nerve cell populations to a similar degree, and some cells may not be affected. The extent of neuronal loss is, perhaps, less extensive than has been assumed previously. No regular or predictable pattern of neuronal degeneration has been established. The loss of neurons is not sufficiently great to account for the reduced ability for control and coordination seen in the nervous system in elderly people.

Loss of Dendrites

Although the number of neurons in most parts of the brain may not be reduced significantly during aging, it has been found that a reduction in the number of dendrites associated with each neuron is a generalized feature of aging. The mechanism of this dendritic loss is unknown, although it has been suggested that the dendritic atrophy begins in the most distal parts of the dendritic branches and gradually works its way toward the cell body of the neuron.[48]

Loss of Synapses

It has been suggested that a typical motor neuron in the spinal cord has perhaps 10,000 synaptic contacts on its surface, of which about 2000 are on its cell body and 8000 are on its dendrites. This does not mean that 10,000 intermediate neurons impinge on the motor neuron; each intermediate neuron tends to make multiple synaptic connections with its target cells. It is evident, then, if the dendritic tree of the neuron is reduced during aging, there will be a loss of synaptic connections with other cells.[49] The number of synaptic connections will also be reduced if degeneration of the terminal branches of axons has occurred.[50] It is not known how many different afferent systems lose their synaptic terminals during senescence.

It is probable that the number of synaptic connections is not static in normal individuals at any age. Synapses may be constantly remodeled during adult life, and the change in the number and distribution of synapses in adulthood may be irregular and may be a reflection of changing functional capacity.[51] In older persons the capacity for remodeling is retained but is usually somewhat reduced. It may be that synapses are lost in the aged brain as a normal part of the turnover process but are less readily replaced.

When new synaptic connections are made some appear to aid in restitution of function, while others oppose this.[52] Misplaced synaptic connections may increase the noise level and decrease the precision of information processing along the abnormal pathways. A theory for the decline of functional capacity of the aged brain is that turnover and cell loss increase the number of inappropriate new connections.[53]

Microscopic Changes in Senescent Neurons

A number of changes are found in the appearance of senescent neurons when these cells are examined under the microscope.

Granules of lipofuscin pigment accumulate in the cell bodies of neurons as a function of age. Traditionally, the pigment has been regarded as resulting from wear and tear processes in those cells with high oxidative activity. Lipofuscin appears to be formed from lysosomal material within the cell. There is no evidence to support the notion that the presence of lipofuscin granules within the cytoplasm will have a detrimental influence on the normal functioning of the cell. Indeed, one of the heaviest accumulations of lipofuscin pigment occurs in the inferior olivary nucleus, which appears to function normally and from which no neurons are lost in senescence.[54]

Evidence of degeneration of the neurofibrils in the cell body is predominant in some types of senile dementia, but such degeneration may also be found in brain cells of persons who have not exhibited symptoms of dementia. It is possible that the stimuli that cause the production of neurofibrillary tangles in cells of the hippocampus, frontotemporal cortex, and reticular formation may cause other degenerative changes in other types of nerve cells.[55] No evidence has been presented to demonstrate that the presence of neurofibrillary tangles causes a decrease in axoplasmic transport, as is often assumed.

Other changes that have been reported—alterations in the Golgi complex, the reduction in ribosome concentration in the endoplasmic reticulum, and the lowered fluid content of the cells—are not restricted to nerve cells but are generalized characteristics of degenerating and senescent cells of all types.

Changes in Nerve Conduction

In the resting state the interior of the nerve cell and its processes are rich in potassium ions and low in sodium ions, whereas on their exterior the concentration of these ions is reversed. Because of this unequal distribution of ions, together with the fact that the membrane in its resting state is much more permeable to potassium than sodium ions, the nerve has a resting potential of approximately 70 mV, the outside being electrically positive with respect to the interior.

A nerve impulse is created by the temporary depolarization of the nerve membrane. Channels in the membrane open up to allow the flow of sodium ions into the cell, with a second set of channels allowing the outward flow of potassium ions from the cell after a slight delay. A wave of depolarization is conducted over the whole surface of the neuron from the point at which it was initially generated. In myelinated nerve fibers the nerve impulse jumps quickly from one node of Ranvier to the next. The conduction velocity of nerve impulses along myelinated fibers is up to 25 times greater than along unmyelinated fibers of similar diameter.

The ionic exchange across the nerve membrane to produce a nerve impulse is a relatively simple mechanism.[56] It is altered little during the aging process. In the elderly there is no significant change in the conduction velocity along a specified portion of a nerve trunk compared to that found in younger adults. In the elderly, as in younger persons, if a reduction in conduction velocity is found, some narrowing of the fiber or some impairment of blood flow to the nerve sheath may be assumed.

Changes in Neurotransmitter Mechanisms

The arrival of a nerve impulse at an axon terminal causes the sudden release of molecules of a transmitter substance from the terminal. The transmitter molecules then diffuse across the fluid-filled gap between the two cells and act on specific receptors on the surface of an adjacent neuron. The electrical activity of the receiving neuron is altered by this action of the transmitter substance. To date, approximately 30 different transmitter substances have been identified; each has a characteristic excitatory or inhibitory effect on the postsynaptic cell.

There are three groups of neurotransmitter substances: (1) those affecting the ionic gate mechanisms, (2) monoamine transmitters, and (3) neuropeptides.

Changes in Ionic Gate Activity. At the nerve–muscle junction and between many neurons in the brain and spinal cord the transmitter substance liberated from the presynaptic cell is acetylcholine. Molecules of acetylcholine are stored in vesicles within the axon terminal. When the nerve impulse arrives at the terminal, calcium ions flow into the depolarized membrane, causing several hundred synaptic vesicles to fuse with the presynaptic membrane. Each vesicle load of acetylcholine causes some 2000 ionic channels to open up in the postsynaptic membrane. Movement of sodium ions into the postsynaptic cell and outflow of potassium ions from the cell will occur.

The acetylcholine molecules in the synaptic gap are rapidly broken down by the enzyme acetylcholinesterase. Most of the channels resulting from this deactivation process will be reabsorbed into the axon terminal of the presynaptic neuron, to be resynthesized back into acetylcholine and re-stored in the terminal for future repeated use. The relative simplicity of this process, combined with the regular resynthesis of acetylcholine molecules, means that this process is not affected by the aging process.[57]

At synapses in the central nervous system where acetylcholine is liberated, a second group of presynaptic neurons terminates. The transmitter liberated from the axon terminals of these presynaptic neurons is γ-aminobutyric acid (GABA). GABA acts on a second set of receptors on the surface of the postsynaptic neuron that opens pores in that membrane that are selectively permeable to negatively charged chloride ions. When these ions pass through the open pores into the postsynaptic cell they increase the voltage across the membrane and temporarily inactivate the cell. Approximately one third of the cells in the central nervous system are thought to use GABA as their neurotransmitter. No GABA-producing neurons terminate at the nerve–muscle interface.

The actions of acetylcholine and GABA upon the postsynaptic cell are complementary. Whether the postsynaptic cell fires or fails to fire when both neurotransmitters are liberated simultaneously is determined by their cumulative effect on the resting potential of the postsynaptic membrane. If the membrane is depolarized because of the stronger excitatory acetylcholine effect, activity will be produced in the postsynaptic neuron, but if the inhibitory action of GABA is greater than the excitatory influence of acetylcholine, the postsynaptic cell will not fire. Like acetylcholine, GABA is rapidly broken down in the synaptic gap and reabsorbed by the presynaptic neuron.

During aging there appears to be a 15 percent reduction in the GABA content of the brain.[58] A reduction in GABA secretion and liberation throughout the nervous system results in some deterioration of fine coordination of activities. When the GABA neurons of the corpus striatum degenerate selectively Huntington's chorea is produced, a condition in which uncontrolled movements are a predominant feature.

Changes in Monoamine Transmitter Activity.   At many synapses the neurotransmitter substance is a monoamine, a substance synthesized within the nerve cell via changes in amino acid molecules absorbed from the bloodstream. For example, molecules of tyrosine are taken into the nerve terminal from the bloodstream and acted upon by enzymes contained in the mitochondria of the axon terminals. In some cells the tyrosine is converted first into dopa and then into dopamine; in other cells the tyrosine is converted into norepinephrine. As the molecules of dopamine and norepinephrine contain a single amino radical, they are termed monoamine transmitters. Other monoamine transmitters have also been identified.

Molecules of monoamine transmitters from the axon terminal interact with specific receptor sites on the postsynaptic membrane. The receptor molecules are coupled in the cell membrane to an enzyme that converts ATP into cyclic adenosine monophospate (cyclic AMP; cAMP). Cyclic AMP then acts on the biochemical machinery of the cell to initiate a further response; cyclic AMP is often termed the "second messenger" substance.

The postsynaptic cell responds to cyclic AMP in two stages. In the first stage depolarization of the membrane of the cell occurs immediately; in the second stage the cell body of the postsynaptic cell may be triggered into synthetic activity. The synthetic activity triggered by this stimulation begins only after some delay but may continue for some time thereafter.

Once the monoamine transmitter has set off the "second messenger" activity its molecules are reabsorbed from the synaptic space back into the axon terminal of the presynaptic neuron. Some are repackaged in synaptic vesicles for repeat use; other molecules are inactivated and destroyed by the enzyme monoamine oxidase in the terminal.[59]

These transmitters are not diffused regularly throughout the brain but are highly localized in discrete centers and pathways. The cell bodies of dopamine-producing cells are located in the substantia nigra of the midbrain, from where some axons project into the corpus striatum, where they play an important part in the control of voluntary movements. Others pass into the forebrain to assist in the control of emotional responses. The cell bodies of the norepinephrine-producing cells are located mostly in the brainstem, from where they pass to the hypothalamus, the cerebellum, and parts of the forebrain where they are important in maintaining arousal and in regulation of mood. The enzymes associated with the metabolism of different transmitter substances are particularly vulnerable to aging changes. If the monoamine pathways degenerate during aging, there will be impairment of motor, emotional, and mood control. Selective degeneration of one or more of these pathways may occur. Where the degeneration selectively affects the dopamine system neurons symptoms of Parkinsonism will develop, while selective degeneration of the norepinephrine pathways will result in depression. The presence of degenerative changes in the monoamine-producing neurons during aging is more pronounced than degenerative changes in other types of neuron.

Changes in Neuropeptide Activity. While transmitters affecting ionic gate mechanisms and the monoamine transmitters are manufactured in the axon terminals of different neurons, a third group of transmitter substances—the neuropeptides—are produced in the cell body.[60] Peptides are chemical substances produced when a number of amino acid molecules are linked together in a particular order to form a single large molecule. The sequence of amino acid components in peptide molecules is fixed, encoded by a gene; thus a strand of DNA in the cell nucleus is required. The genetic encoding mechanism in the nucleus is transcribed onto a strand of messenger RNA, which carries the code to the ribosome. Ribosomes in the cell body are the sites at which the peptide synthesis occurs. The original peptide molecule synthesized by the ribosomes is very large; enzymes in the cell body cleave the larger peptide strand into a number of shorter chains. Different groups of nerve cells contain different enzyme systems, and thus the transmitter neuropeptide substance produced varies according to the enzyme system of the cell. Neurotransmitters produced in this way include P-substance, endorphin, and ACTH.

Once the neuropeptides have been synthesized in the cell body they must be transported along the whole length of the axon to its terminals. Those substances that are relatively small may be carried in the fast-transport mechanism of the neuron; the larger neuropeptides will be carried in the slow-transport mechanism. The action of cyclic AMP as the "second messenger" in the cell body will stimulate the production of the neuropeptide and its transport to the axon terminals. The effect of stimulation, triggering the production of neuropeptides in the cell body and the release of the substance at the terminals, may continue for minutes or hours. The mechanisms involved in the encoding, synthesis, transport, storage, liberation, and inactivation of neuropeptides are obviously more complex than those involved in other types of neurotransmitters; as a result these mechanisms are more affected by the normal aging process.

P-substance is a chain of amino acids produced in, and liberated by, nerve cells along the pain pathways. Ribosomes in some of the cells in the posterior root ganglion produce molecules of P-substance, which are transported throughout the neuron. The generation of a nerve impulse along the pain fibers causes P-substance molecules to be liberated from the axon terminals of these fibers in the substantia gelatinosa. The second-stage neurons in the lateral spinothalamic tract, which pass upward in the central nervous system to the thalamus, liberate further amounts of P-substance in the thalamus. Reuptake of P-substance from the synaptic cleft into the presynaptic terminal is a slow process compared with the rate of uptake of monoamine transmitters. While molecules of P-substance remain, pain sensation will persist.

Another neuropeptide substance, similar in chemical composition to morphine, is liberated from other axon terminals in the proximity of synapses along the pain pathway. This substance is known as endorphin. Endorphin appears to have an action on the axon terminals of the pain nerve fibers by inhibiting the ability of those fibers to release P-substance. This will result in reducing the number of pain impulses to the brain.

Normally the secretion and activity of P-substance and endorphin is well coordinated. During the aging process the production and activity of one or both of these substances may be impaired. In some elderly people a generalized reduction of sensory activity may occur, largely owing to a raised threshold level of stimulation being required to trigger activity in the sensory nerves. In this situation, and when the pain pathways selectively degenerate, this sensitivity to painful stimulation will be reduced. In other persons selective degeneration of the endorphin-producing neurons will result in increased sensitivity to pain and possibly the development of certain types of chronic pain state. Acupuncture is thought to produce its pain-relieving effect largely through stimulation of increased secretion of endorphins. Older persons are less responsive to treatment by acupuncture, probably as the result of a decreased ability to produce endorphins.[61]

Commentary

Many losses associated with advanced aging (reduced sensibility, coordination, cognition, and adaptability) had been assumed to be due to loss of nerve tissue. The reduced level of nervous system function in the elderly is better explained in terms of biochemical changes that take place in neurons with advanced age. It appears that the three groups of neurotransmitter substances are each affected in a different way by the normal aging process. The neurotransmitters that affect the ionic gate mechanism are GABA and acetylcholine. The relative simplicity of the acetylcholine mechanism of activity means that this process is not affected in a significant way by the aging process. The presence of GABA, a neurotransmitter found in the central nervous system is reduced by 15 percent with advanced age. The clinical implication is a deterioration of fine coordination of movement. The monoamine transmitters (dopamine and norepinephrine) impact the body in highly specific centers in the brain. A dysfunction in the monoamine transmitter activity can result in an alteration of mood, emotion, or motor control. The most common clinical signs are Parkinson disease and depression. During advanced aging there appear to be more degenerative changes found in the monoamine-producing neurons than in other types of neurons.

The third group of transmitter substances, the neuropeptides (P-substance, endorphin, and ATCH), involve a complex mechanism of encoding, synthesis, transport, storage, liberation, and inactivation. The production of neuropeptides is more complex than that for the other two groups of neurotransmitters, and it is therefore more affected by the normal aging process. Clinically, since P-substance and endorphin activity are impaired, the result is an altered sensory response to stimuli. The result of a decrease in P-substance production can be an overall decrease in sensory responsiveness. The decrease in P-substance production results in an increased threshold level for stimulation and therefore a decreased sensitivity to pain. If the distortion is a decrease in production and activity of endorphin, the patient will be increasingly sensitive to pain. In either situation, there is a need for special clinical procedures for the management of pain in the elderly and prevention of accidents related to an altered pain threshold.

IMPLICATIONS OF BIOLOGIC CHANGES OF AGING ON EXERCISE PROGRAMS FOR THE ELDERLY

In development of exercise programs for the elderly, consideration must be given to the development of coordination, endurance, strength, and power. The exercise program must have a clear functional goal relevant to the patient.

Coordination

There is a significant loss of coordination noted in the elderly, although whether this is due to disuse, lack of fitness, normal aging, or a combination of these factors is difficult to determine. The loss of coordination with advanced age need not affect self-care capacity. The following discussion is directed toward management of patients experiencing changes in coordination due to the interaction of disuse, lack of fitness, normal aging, and/or pathology.

A decrease of coordination is noted in early adult life and continues progressively from that time. The performance of an efficient, skilled movement that is properly coordinated depends on two factors: avoidance of unnecessary muscle activity and an almost perfect replication of the activity on succeeding attempts.

When a movement is performed in an uncoordinated fashion a considerable amount of unnecessary muscle activity is performed. Muscles not required to function at all in the activity are brought into action, and those muscles essential to the performance of the activity work more than necessary. As a training effect is produced, the amount of unnecessary activity is progressively reduced.

When an untrained subject makes repeated attempts to perform an activity, considerable variation occurs between one attempt and the next in the way the movement is executed. In a trained subject the degree of variation is reduced; a well-trained subject is able to accurately reproduce the movement on succeeding attempts.

Both reduction of extraneous muscle action and perfect replication of movements result from the development of new patterns of nerve activity in the central nervous system. The training of coordination involves a training of central nervous system activity. The synaptic resistance along the frequently used pathways in the central nervous system is reduced, thereby facilitating repeated performance of that activity at a later time.

In dealing with geriatric patients and others with a low exercise tolerance (as measured by cardiopulmonary response) it is preferable to commence the rehabilitation program with attempts to improve the efficiency of those functions the patient is able to perform before progressing to training of new activities, the development of endurance, and improvement in strength and power of muscle contraction.

In the elderly there is not only an overall slowing down of performance but also greater irregularity and unevenness. Practice brings greater uniformity of performance, but some reorganization may be needed to distribute the older person's resources more effectively over the whole task. The therapist therefore should not limit activity to patching up of an existing performance but should consider reorganizing the whole pattern of behavior. Skilled performance is not merely the sum of its component parts; component parts may be acquired individually, but they become transformed when they are incorporated into the large serial organization.[62]

Retraining of coordination in older persons will be more successful if it is gradual; if the trainees can approach the task in their own way at their own speed; if mistakes in performance can be avoided, especially in the early stages of learning; and if the activity is valued by the learner. The therapist needs to recognize that the older person's unique perceptual and cognitive processes make the approach to retraining very different from that employed with younger patients (see Chapter 3).

Endurance

An endurance exercise is characterized by the performance of an activity over a period of time with moderate loading of the working muscles. An increase in endurance occurs when a person can continue to perform a given activity for a longer period of time without fatigue. In other words, there has been an increase in the aerobic capacity.

During activity the different types of muscle fiber are recruited in a regular order; the slow oxidative type I fibers are recruited first, the fast oxidative/glycolytic type IIa fibers are recruited next, and the fast glycolytic type IIb fibers are recruited last. It is evident, then, that recruitment of type IIa and type IIb fibers will only occur if the load applied is sufficiently high.

Improvement in the oxidative enzyme and myoglobin content of type I and type IIb fibers have been reported within 2 to 3 days of commencement of a program of endurance exercises. The degree of improvement and the rate at which aerobic capacity improves depend on the amount of loading applied. In young adults the performance of an activity that loads the muscle to 90 percent of its capacity for 15 minutes three times weekly over a 2 month period is said to lead to a 15 percent increase in maximum oxygen uptake. A similar degree of improvement over the same period with 60 percent loading requires 1 to 2 hours of exercise three times weekly; with 30 percent loading, 1 to 2 hours of daily exercise would be necessary.

In older subjects improvement is likely to be slower and might occur to a lesser degree.[63] The effects of endurance exercise programs for the elderly that have been reported in the literature are variable. It is possible that in those programs that have not led to reported physiologic changes either the loading was insufficient or the length of the training program was too short; the former appears more likely. It is reasonable to expect that the endurance capacity of all persons, regardless of age, can be increased providing that the loading is sufficiently heavy and providing that the program is continued over a sufficiently long period.

Endurance training not only produces an increase in the oxidative enzyme content of type I and type IIa fibers but also results in an increase in the density of the capillary bed in the working muscles. Exchange of materials between the blood and tissue fluid across the capillary wall is facilitated.

Endurance training for young subjects involves total body activity; many muscles are used in the performance of that activity. When the muscles contract, blood is pumped into the venous side of the circulatory system. An increased venous return to the heart is produced, resulting in an increase in both stroke volume and heart rate. Over time, a training effect on the heart will be observed: the performance of a given exercise leads to a smaller increase in heart rate.

The cardiac reserve in elderly persons is less than in younger subjects. The performance of even light general activity by an old person may result in an increase in cardiac rate to an undesirably high level. It is essential that the heart rate be monitored during the activity to avoid this.

In order to avoid undue strain on the heart, activity restricted to one part of the body may have to be the starting point for general exercise in severely debilitated individuals. In general, lower limb activities place less strain on the heart than equivalent exercise to the upper limbs. While the performance of light general exercise may be useful in producing a cardiac training effect over a period of time, no significant effect will be produced with the working muscles unless the exercise meets the criteria of loading and duration described earlier. When establishing an endurance training program for debilitated elderly patients it may be desirable to begin with a regimen of upper and lower limb *functional* endurance exercises on alternate days, with progression to general body activity only after some improvement in the cardiac reserve has been developed.

The risk that inappropriate exercise may precipitate cardiac arrest or ventricular fibrillation is small. For men 65 to 70 years old the risk has been estimated at 1 in 27,000, while risks for elderly women would be approximately one third those for males.[64] As the risk would appear to be greatest in those persons with a highly competitive "type A" personality, the chance of this problem in geriatric patients is extremely remote. In dealing with geriatric patients, fear of heart attacks by either the patient or the therapist often precludes the development of an effective training program.

The initial exercise regimen should be planned to keep the maximum heart rate in older persons below 130 beats per minute. For most geriatric patients fast walking readily raises the heart rate to this level. In the early weeks of training approximately equal distances (400 m) can be covered by fast and slow walking over a 30-minute period. This type of program for elderly people has been shown to result in a 20 percent gain in maximum oxygen uptake over a period of 21 weeks.[63] The largest increase was produced in those subjects who followed a high-intensity/high-frequency exercise regimen. These subjects also showed a faster recovery of heart rate following submaximum and maximum exercise efforts. However, slowing of the resting pulse rate is not found when older people undergo conditioning.[65] Those subjects who show an improvement in physical fitness also show decreases in ST abnormalities on EKG records; this is considered attributable to a reduction of the heart rate when a given workload is applied[66] (see Chapter 8).

Muscle Strength

Strength involves the development of maximum tension in the muscle during muscle contraction. To a certain extent this may be a result of an increased proportion of muscle fibers within the muscle belly recruited during a maximum effort. The degree of improvement from this mechanism is comparatively small; untrained normal individuals recruit up to 35 percent of the total number of fibers, while trained subjects may be able to increase this proportion to 40 percent. In older persons the proportion of fibers that may be voluntarily recruited is considerably lower.

True hypertrophy of the muscle fibers (i.e., an increase in the amount of contractile protein contained within the muscle fiber) will occur only if the muscle is caused to contract against a heavy resistance.[67] Progressive recruitment of different types of muscle fiber will occur as the resistance is increased, with the type IIb fast glycolytic fibers brought into action only when heavy loads have to be overcome.

Isometric exercise is most effective for developing the tension within the muscle that is required to stimulate the production of actomyosin by the muscle ribosomes. At first, maximum tension within the muscle should be developed slowly during the isometric contraction; later this can be speeded up. Static holding of the contraction against an increasing resistance should be practiced. *It should be recognized that until a certain degree of coordination and endurance exists, or has been built up, the results of isometric training tend to be ineffective.* Isometric exercise programs for the elderly are often ineffective due to inadequate loading of the contracting muscles.

The elderly take longer to show improvement in strength than younger persons, a reflection of the increased difficulty of actomyosin synthesis in the muscles of older persons. The potential does remain, however, for hypertrophy to be produced in the muscle fibers of older persons as the result of properly conducted isometric training programs. If the hypertrophy is to be maintained in an elderly person it is necessary for isometric exercises to be continued on a regular basis. In younger persons the hypertrophy tends to be maintained for up to 2 months if the exercise program is stopped, but this is not the case with older individuals.[68]

For maximum development of strength, exercise at very high intensity or force levels relative to the maximum is required. Although bouts of this intensive exercise should be repeated, the number of repetitions need only be low; two or three bouts of six to ten repetitions performed once a day is usually considered sufficient.[69]

In those elderly persons in whom muscle weakness is produced through functional denervation rather than simple disuse, the application of high loads to the contracting muscles may result in some further weakening of those muscles. Overwork weakness has been reported particularly in muscles denervated by poliomyelitis[70] and muscular dystrophy.[71] Muscles that have been partially denervated as a result of aging processes might demonstrate a similar overwork weakness, although this has never been reported in the literature.

Power Development

As a means of increasing power—rate of working—isokinetic types of exercise are the most effective. Certain devices—e.g., the Cybex apparatus—have been designed for isokinetic training. The apparatus can be adjusted to allow movements to be performed at various speeds, with the angular velocity of the movement remaining constant throughout the whole range once the controls have been set. The patient exerts maximum effort throughout the movement.

Special equipment is not necessary to train isokinetic activity. When using manual resistance, whether to isolated or pattern movements, therapists tend to vary the resistance they apply in different parts of the range in such a way that the movement is performed smoothly. It is evident that therapists have used the concept of isokinetic training in their rehabilitation exercise programs quite unknowingly (proprioceptive neuromuscular facilitation).

Progression in the development of power is made by requiring the patient to perform a given exercise more frequently within a given time or, alternatively, by requiring that the same number of contractions be completed within a fixed period even though the resistance to the movement has been increased.

Only if the particular deficits are properly identified and if appropriate strategies to deal with these are devised can significant functional improvement be expected. The lower exercise tolerance of older persons makes it necessary to plan each part of the program with extreme care, so that maximum effectiveness is obtained.

HORMONAL CONTROL MECHANISMS AND AGING

In a small number of neurons in the central nervous system the peptide produced within the cell body of the neuron is ACTH. Liberation of ACTH from the axon terminals of these neurons produces different effects on different groups of postsynaptic cells. ACTH and a number of other peptide transmitter substances that have been identified are substances also produced outside the nervous system by cells of the endocrine system. When produced by endocrine cells, these substances are termed hormones.

At neuron-to-neuron connections the transmitter molecules are produced in moderate amounts and will be released from the presynaptic cell only through the axon terminals. The small amount of transmitter substance liberated from the axon terminal is rapidly deactivated at the release site. The effect of release of neurotransmitters is limited to a very localized area for only a short period of time.

Movement of molecules between capillaries and extracellular spaces in the central nervous system is more difficult than in other tissues. Nerve cells have become more sensitive than other types of cells to their immediate chemical environment to facilitate a variety of specific transmitter mechanisms; thus the nerve cells need to be protected from the presence of stray molecules of other materials that may appear by chance in the area. Such protection is obtained by increased resistance of the capillary walls to the passage of many substances contained in the blood plasma. The passage of food-derived peptide molecules across the capillary wall, in particular, would obviously grossly upset the peptide-controlled neurotransmitter mechanisms.[58]

The capillary wall thickening is achieved partly by a thickening of the basement membrane of the epithelial cells that form the capillary wall and partly as the result of glial cell activity. The glial cells are connective tissue cells responsible for producing the connective tissue packing material for the nerve cells and their fibers. The protein glial membranes that are produced contain finer fibers than those contained in other connective tissues. The presence of a glial membrane around the small blood vessels and capillaries in the brain produces the so-called blood–brain barrier, which reduces the possibility of stray peptide movement.

During aging the glial cells often become somewhat more active, with the result that the glial membrane is thickened. If this should occur the passage of materials across this blood–brain barrier becomes still more difficult. The volume of the extracellular space will be reduced.

Although these changes make it less likely that the nerve cell function is affected by diffusion of stray peptide molecules, passage of other materials across the membrane necessary for the continued proper functioning of the nerve cells is also made more difficult. It is possible that at those sites in the brain at which selective neuronal degeneration has been demonstrated, the degeneration may be linked, at least in part, to thickening of the blood–brain barrier at these locations.

While all neuron-to-neuron connections in the brain are protected by the blood–brain barrier, some nerve connections are made with cells outside the nervous system. Such connections form the neuroendocrine system.[72] Connections from the hypothalamus to the posterior lobe of the pituitary gland belong to this system. The cells in the posterior lobe of the pituitary gland lie outside the blood–brain barrier. Stimulation of cells in this area will result in liberation of peptide molecules from the cells. These molecules will pass into the bloodstream as it flows through the area.

Cells in the true endocrine glands—anterior lobe of the pituitary gland, the thyroid gland, etc.—respond to stimuli from chemicals in the blood flowing through the gland rather than from chemical stimulation from direct neurotransmitter activity. The exercise of some control of activity in the anterior lobe of the pituitary gland by the hypothalamus is not through direct neuronal connections. Neurohormones are liberated from nerve endings in the hypothalamus, enter the pituitary portal vessels, and then pass directly into the anterior lobe of the pituitary where they help regulate its secretions.[73]

As the result of specific patterns of neural activity, neurotransmitter substances are liberated at particular sites to produce localized changes for short periods of time. To complement this, the endocrine system of the body provides for simultaneous regulation and coordination of activities to modify the structure and function of distant organs and tissues of the body over longer periods. This is achieved through the action of chemical substances secreted by certain collections of cells and transported throughout the body via the blood and lymph. Normally, the activity of many endocrine glands is finely balanced and highly coordinated. In the elderly the coordination is increasingly disrupted.

Much of this disruption is the result of the body's reaction to increasing stress. When a person is exposed to stress—whether physical, psychologic, sociologic, economic, or emotional—changes take place in the body in an attempt to deal with the stress. Many of these changes involve a shift away from the normal endocrine balance. Selye referred to this reaction as the general adaptation syndrome (GAS), and he divided the response into three distinct phases: the alarm reaction, the stage of resistance, and the stage of exhaustion.[74]

Aging is a period of chronic and increasing stress. The development of the GAS in elderly persons differs somewhat from the reaction in younger subjects. In the alarm reaction and stage of resistance the degree of response tends to be much reduced. As the result of chronic stress from multiple causes the body's defense mechanisms may not be able to cope, and the stage of exhaustion ensues. In the stage of exhaustion physiologic responses become increasingly unpredictable;

they may be greater or less than the usual responses in younger persons, or may be opposite in direction—paradoxical—to the normal reaction.

The physiology of older persons should not be viewed as a simple continuation of those processes operating in younger individuals. It needs to be recognized that the responses of the elderly may differ both quantitatively and qualitatively from the reactions of young adults due to varying patterns of change and degeneration in the various mechanisms involved in maintaining the body's homeostasis. Similarly, the signs and symptoms of disease exhibited by older persons may be different from those presented by younger persons suffering from the same disease. A better knowledge of the biologic changes of aging not only will enable physical therapists to understand the limitations of their older clients more fully but will enable them to plan more effective treatment programs.

REFERENCES

1. Goldberg B, Green H: Collagen synthesis on polyribosomes of cultured mammalian fibroblasts. J Mol Biol 26:1–18, 1975.
2. Gross J: Organization and disorganization of collagen. Biophys J 4:63–77, 1964.
3. Chapman JA, et al: Assembly of collagen fibrils. Fed Proc 25:1811–1814, 1966.
4. Ramachandrau GN, Saisakharan V: Refinement of the structure of collagen. Biochem Biophys Acta 109:314–316, 1965.
5. Vais A, Anasey J: Modes of intermolecular cross linking in mature insoluble collagen. J Biol Chem 240:3899–3908, 1965.
6. Barnes MJ: Function of ascorbic acid in collagen metabolism. Ann NY Acad Sci 258:264–277, 1975.
7. Ehrlich HP, Hunt TK: Effects of cortisone and vitamin A on wound healing. Ann Surg 167:324–328, 1968.
8. King AL: In: Tissue Elasticity, ed. Remington JW, Waverly Press, Baltimore, Md., 1957.
9. Meyer K, et al: Mucopolysaccharides of costal cartilage. Science 128:896, 1958.
10. Lehmann JF, et al: Effect of therapeutic temperatures on tendon extensibility. Arch Phys Med Rehabil 50:481–485, 1970.
11. Ryan GB, et al: Myofibroblasts in human granulation tissue. Hum Pathol 5:55–67, 1974.
12. Kaplan D, Mayer K: Distribution of alkaline phosphatase. Nature 183:1262–1263, 1959.
13. Cailliet R: Mechanisms of joints. In: Arthritis and Physical Medicine, ed. Licht S. Waverly Press, Baltimore, Md., 1969.
14. Atkinson PJ: Structural aspects of aging bone. Gerontologia 15:171–173, 1973.
15. Lutwak L: Continuing need for dietary calcium throughout life. Geriatrics 29:177–178, 1974.
16. Bargel US: Osteoporosis. Grune and Stratton, New York, 1970.
17. Mundy GR, et al: Evidence for the secretion of an osteoclast stimulating factor in myeloma. N Engl J Med: 291:1041–1046, 1974.
18. Berlyne GM, et al: The aetiology of senile osteoporosis. Q J Med 44:505–521, 1975.
19. Storey E: Bone changes associated with cortisone administration in the rat. Br J Exp Pathol 41:207–213, 1960.

20. Towne EA: Electron microscopic evidence of altering osteocytic-osteoclastic and osteoplastic activity in peri-lacunar walls of aging mice. Connect Tissue Res 1:221–230, 1972.
21. Burstone MS: Histochemical demonstration of acid phosphatase activity in osteoclasts. J Histochem Cytochem 7:39–41, 1959.
22. Ham AW, Harris R: Repair and transplantation in bone. In: Biology and Physiology of Bone, ed. Bourne GH. Academic Press, New York, 1971.
23. Newton-John HF, Morgan DB: The loss of bone with age, osteoporosis and fractures. Clin Orthop 71:229–252, 1970.
24. Khairi MRA, Johnston CG: What we know and don't know about bone loss in the elderly. Geriatrics 33:67–76, Nov 1978.
25. Issekutz B, et al: Effect of prolonged bed rest on urinary calcium output. J Appl Physiol 21:1013–1020, 1966.
26. Geiser M, Trueta J: Muscle action, bone rarefaction and bone formation. J Bone Jt Surg 40B:282–311, 1968.
27. Kumar S, et al: Bone marrow pressure and bone strength. Acta Orthop Scand 50:507–512, 1979.
28. Bassett CAL: Effect of force on skeletal tissues. In: Physiological Basis of Rehabilitation Medicine, ed. Downey JA and Darling RC. Saunders, Philadelphia, Pa., 1971.
29. Nordin BEC: Calcium balance and calcium requirement in spinal osteoporosis. Am J Clin Nutr 10:384–390, 1962.
30. Exton-Smith AW: The management of osteoporosis. Proc R Soc Med 69:931–934, 1976.
31. Experimental biomechanics of intervertebral disc rupture through a vertebral body. J Neurosurg 30:134–139, 1969.
32. Frost HM: The Laws of Bone Structure. C. C Thomas, Springfield, Ill., 1964.
33. Aaron JE, et al: Frequency of osteomalacia and osteoporosis in fractures of the proximal femur. Lancet 1:229–233, 1974.
34. Yiengst MJ, et al: Age changes in the chemical composition of muscle and liver in the rat. J Gerontol 14:400–404, 1959.
35. Anderson F: Practical Management of the Elderly, 3rd ed. Backwell, Oxford, 1976.
36. Drahota Z, Gutmann E: Long term regulatory influence of the nervous system on some metabolic differences in muscles of different function. Physiol Bohemoslov 12:339–348, 1963.
37. Finch CE: Enzyme activity, gene function, and aging in mammals. Exp Gerontol 7:53–67, 1972.
38. Tomanek RJ, Woo JK: Compensatory hypertrophy of the plantaris muscle in relation to age. J Gerontol 25:23–29, 1970.
39. Campbell MJ, et al: Physiological changes in ageing muscles. J Neurol Neurosurg Psychiatry 36:174–182, 1973.
40. Tomonage M: Histochemical and ultrastructural changes in senile human skeletal muscles. J Am Gerontol Soc 25:125–131, 1977.
41. Vrolova G: Factors determining the speed of contraction of striated muscle. J Physiol 185:17–18, 1966.
42. Walder DN: Vascular pathways in skeletal muscle. In: Circulation in Skeletal Muscle, ed. Hudlicka O. Pergamon, Oxford, 1968.
43. Ordy JM, Brizzee KR: Neurobiology of Aging. Plenum, New York, 1975.
44. Himwich HE: Biochemistry of the nervous system in relation to the process of aging.

In: The Process of Aging in the Nervous System, ed. Birren JE, et al. C. C Thomas, Springfield, Ill., 1959.

45. Corsellis JAN: Some observations in the Purkinje cell population and on brain volume in human aging. In: Neurobiology of Aging, ed. Terry RD, Gershon S. Raven Press, New York, 1976.

46. Ball MJ: Neuronal loss, neurofibrillary tangles and granulovacuolar degeneration in the hippocampus with aging and dementia. Acta Neuropathol 37:111–118, 1976.

47. Konigsmark BW, Murphy EA: Neuronal populations in the human brain. Nature 228:1335–1336, 1970.

48. Vaughan DW: Age related deterioration of pyramidal cell basal dendrites in the rat auditory cortex. J Comp Neurol 171:501–516, 1977.

49. Nauta WJH, Feirtag M: Organization of the brain. Sci Am 241:88–111, Sep 1979.

50. Bondareff W: Synaptic atrophy in the senescent hippocampus. Mech Age Dev 9:163–171, 1979.

51. Sotelo C, Palay SL: Altered axons and axon terminals in the lateral vestibular nucleus of the rat—Possible example of remodelling. Lab Invest 25:653–671, 1976.

52. Schneider GE: Synaptic remodelling. Neuropsychologia 17:557–583, 1979.

53. Cotman CW: Synaptic structure and plasticity. In: Biological Mechanisms of Aging, ed. Schimke RJ. National Institutes of Health, Bethesda, Md., 1981.

54. Brody H: Aging in the vertebrate brain. In: Development and Aging of the Nervous System, Academic Press, New York, 1973.

55. Wisniewski WM, Terry RD: Morphology of the aging brain: Human and animal. Prog Brain Res 40:167–186, 1973.

56. Keynes R: Ion channels in the nerve cell membrane. Sci Am 240:126–135, March 1979.

57. Hollander J, Barrows CH: Enzymatic studies in senescent rodent brain. J Gerontol 23:174–179, 1968.

58. Iversen LL: The chemistry of the brain. Sci Am 241:134–149, Sep 1979.

59. McGeer EG, McGeer PL: Age changes in the human for some enzymes associated with metabolism of catecholamines, GABA, and acetylcholine. In: Neurobiology of Aging, eds. Ordy JM, Brizzee KE. Plenum, New York, 1975.

60. Bloom FE: Neuropeptides. Sci Am 245:148–169, Oct 1981.

61. Sodipo JOA: Therapeutic acupuncture for chronic pain. Pain 7:359–365, Dec 1979.

62. Bromley DB: The Psychology of Human Aging. Pelican, Harmondsworth, 1966.

63. Sidney KH, Shephard RJ: Maximum and sub-maximum exercise tests in men and women in the seventh, eighth, and ninth decades of life. J Appl Physiol 43:280–287, 1977.

64. Shephard RJ: Physical Activity and Aging. Croom Helm, Chicago, 1978.

65. Stamford BA: Physiological effects of training upon institutionalized geriatric men. J Gerontol 27:451–455, 1972.

66. Costill DL, et al: Effects of physical training in men with coronary heart disease. Med Sci Sports 6:95–100, 1974.

67. Hansen JW: The training effect of repeated isometric muscle contractions. Int Z Angew Physiol 18:474–477, 1961.

68. Karlsson J, et al: Muscle lactate, ATP, and CP levels during exercise after physical training in men. J Appl Physiol 33:199–203, Aug 1972.

69. Hislop HJ: Quantitative changes in human muscular strength during isometric exercise. J Am Phys Ther Assoc 43:21–38, 1963.

70. Bennett RL, Knowlton GC: Overwork weakness in partially denervated skeletal muscles. Clin Orthop 12:22–28, 1958.

71. Johnson EWJ, Braddon R: Overwork weakness in facio-scapulo-humeral muscular dystrophy. Arch Phys Med Rehabil 52:333–336, 1971.
72. Everitt AV, Burgess JA: Hypothalamus, Pituitary, and Aging. C. C Thomas, Springfield, Ill., 1976.
73. Harris GW: Neural Control of the Pituitary Gland. Arnold, London, 1955.
74. Selye H, Prioreski B: Stress in relation to aging and disease. In: Hypothalamus, Pituitary, and Aging, eds. Everitt AV, Burgess JA. C. C Thomas, Springfield, Ill., 1976.

3 | Older Adult Learning

David A. Peterson
Rosemary A. Orgren

The process of physical therapy intervention involves evaluation followed by planning of a program of therapeutic care to accomplish one or more specific goals. The process of rehabilitation can be described as a process of relearning tasks/movements and associated attitudes. Rehabilitation can also involve habilitation or the learning of a task/movement and the related attitude that has never been previously mastered. Rehabilitation and physical therapy care for the elderly need an examination of the specific instructional strategies that facilitate learning for persons in their later years.

Educational intervention in the lives of older adults has been a subject of rapidly increasing interest over the past ten years. This interest originates not only from a recognition that individuals have learning needs at every age, but also from an appreciation of the plasticity of human intelligence and the conviction that people can continue to grow and change throughout life. Literature on the intelligence and learning abilities of older persons, while sometimes inconclusive, tends to support the convictions that intellectual aging is modifiable and that learning at any age is possible and valuable. Further, it suggests that there may be specific instructional strategies that facilitate learning in later years.

Any comprehensive discussion of how to help older adults learn, however, must be more than merely prescriptive; an understanding of the derivation of useful strategies is equally important. Such basic knowledge will assist therapists to use these strategies more successfully and perhaps guide them in generating innovative strategies of their own. This chapter consequently both offers practical suggestions to facilitate the learning of older adults and describes the foundation of these ideas in psychologic and educational research.

The chapter is divided into two major sections: discussion of research on older adult intelligence and learning performance and the implications of this research for improving care for the elderly. Although a certain amount of overlap exists between these two areas, they are sufficiently distinct to indicate that such a separation is reasonable. The chapter proceeds from the more abstract concerns of research studies on older adult intelligence to the more practical application of instructional strategies for dealing with older people.

INTELLIGENCE

Many studies have attempted to determine the intelligence of individuals and to ascertain if change typically occurs in this attribute over the course of the lifespan. The literature describing these findings offers a massive accumulation of data on the basic questions. However, definitive answers are not yet available, and researchers still differ on some points concerning the relationship of intelligence and age. A review of these studies provides insight into the intellectual potential and performance of middle-aged and older persons and indicates several significant implications for those who would provide instruction and training to persons in these age groups.

The Meaning of Intelligence

As with most fundamental concepts, intelligence is difficult to define. It is usually considered to consist of the cognitive capacity of the individual, ability to learn, facility at manipulating and understanding common and unique items. This cognitive potential is impossible to measure directly; thus all research on intelligence has inferred the underlying traits of an individual by measuring performance in a number of settings. Performance and innate ability (potential) are not necessarily synonymous, since numerous factors (health, perceptual acuity, motivation, cultural factors) can affect performance. The potential of elderly patients coming to physical therapy can be greatly underestimated because they usually manifest problems with health, distortion of perceptual acuity, and depression and other emotional stress, which generally affects motivation. Thus intelligence quotient (IQ), the performance measure, may closely approximate the ceiling potential of the individual or may greatly underestimate it.

Likewise, high IQ scores do not assure an individual career success, do not indicate social or vocational competence, and may not lead to adaptation to the society or any particular role. IQ historically was developed as a means to predict success in educational endeavors. Since it deals with cognitive abilities and since these are closely related to any learning enterprise, it has proved to be a fairly relible indicator of performance in an educational setting. It is also very useful in estimating success in employment that has high educational prerequisites. However, even for the highly educated there are many areas of life in which such learning is not particularly relevant. In these areas (interpersonal relations, adjustment, physical strength, beauty, commitment, self-esteem, motivation, or wisdom) other variables may prove to be substantially more powerful determinants of success than intelligence. Thus intelligence should be considered as an important attribute of each individual, but high or low scores do not automatically determine the quality of performance that can be expected from that individual.

Although intelligence is a singular noun, most psychologists would agree that there is no single entity that can be thought of as "intelligence." It is probably more accurate to think of "intelligences," which each individual has and which can be measured in a variety of ways. One concept of intelligence that has received wide acceptance over the past 15 years is that of fluid and crystallized intelligence.[1] Crystallized intelligence depends upon sociocultural influences; it involves the ability to perceive relations, to engage in formal reasoning, and to understand the intellectual and cultural heritage. It is measured through culture-specific items such as number facility, verbal comprehension, and general information. Thus the amount the individual learns, the diversity and complexity of the environment, the openness to new information, and the extent of formal learning opportunities are likely to be influential in the score of the individual. In general, crystallized intelligence continues to grow slowly throughout adulthood as the individual acquires increased information and develops an understanding of the relationships of diverse facts and constructs. Continued acculturation through self-directed learning and education can encourage the growth of crystallized intelligence even after the age of 60.[2]

Fluid intelligence, on the other hand, is not closely associated with acculturation. It is generally considered to be independent of instruction or environment and depends more upon the genetic endowment of the individual. It consists of the ability to perceive complex relations, use short-term memory, create concepts, and undertake abstract reasoning. Items included in tests of fluid intelligence are memory span, inductive reasoning, and figural relations, all of which are assumed to be unresponsive to training or exercise. (One must be careful not to confuse training or exercise in performing on *tests* that measure these attributes with training or exercise in the attributes themselves.) Fluid intelligence involves those items that are the most neurophysiologic in nature and are generally assumed to decline after the individual reaches maturity. However, the decline through middle age is quite small; at middle age scores on fluid intelligence tasks are no lower than scores in midadolescence.[2]

Intellectual Changes Over the Lifespan

The earliest studies of adult intelligence showed an increase in IQ until the late teens or early twenties and then a slow decline throughout the rest of the adult years. These studies used a cross-sectional design that tested people of several ages and then compared the scores of younger people with those of other persons who were older. The differences in the scores were assumed to be related to age. Later studies have used longitudinal designs in which the same persons were tested at various points over the lifespan, with changes compared so that trends in intellectual performance could be observed. These studies have reported a somewhat different pattern of change, with less decline occurring and with IQ increasing in some cases.

Before examining these trends, however, we must consider once again the great individual differences that exist in intellectual functioning. Any general description of the relationship of age to intellectual change will obscure some of the variation observable in a large population. Thus knowledge of the age of an individual is insufficient to estimate whether that person is intelligent or not, or whether because of age any individual has suffered such decline to be no longer capable of learning or functioning successfully. Age does have some effect on intelligence, but it does not override many other influencing factors.

Botwinick[3] has described the "classic aging pattern of intelligence." Over the adult portion of the lifespan verbal abilities decline very little if at all, while psychomotor abilities decline earlier and to a greater extent. Thus on the WAIS (Wechsler Adult Intelligence Scale) the verbal subtests show virtual stability throughout the years from age 20 to 60, while the performance subtests show decline from the late 20s on. After age 65 to 70 decline in both areas increases but does not reach a point where the individual is incompetent. Eisdorfer et al.[4] reported that this pattern holds for men and women, black and white adults, individuals from various economic strata, and persons in both mental hospitals and the community. These findings are consistent with the notion that crystallized intelligence is maintained over the adult lifespan, while fluid intelligence declines. The decline in fluid intelligence and the growth in crystallized intelligence are assumed to approximately balance out, so that the loss of biologic potential is offset by the wisdom, experience, and knowledge that the older adult has acquired. Stability of intellectual performance over the greatest part of the typical lifespan would appear to be normal, and persons in their 50s should have maintained learning ability equal to what they had in their 20s *when they can control the pace.* Although ability may begin to fall off between the ages of 60 and 70, the tasks that become most difficult are those that are fast-paced, unusual, and complex.[2]

The amount of deficit that occurs after age 70, however, is unclear. Although a fairly sharp decline is typically shown, this may be caused by what has been called "terminal drop." This phenomenon, first reported by Riegel and Riegel,[5] is a decline in the IQ scores of individuals a few years prior to death and is thought to be caused by physiologic deterioration. For some reason, intellectual functioning appears to be one means of predicting approaching death. If the older sample in any study included a preponderance of persons who were nearing death, their IQ scores would indicate a substantial decline compared to younger persons; however, this may be traced to their nearness to death and not to some other change that occurs around age 70. Thus intellectual decline that results at this time may be primarily caused by the approach of death and not some cognitive factor. Increased medical treatment, preventive health care, and improved public health may prolong the healthy portion of life and consequently extend the period in which intelligence remains basically stable.

Schaie[6] has suggested an alternative view of lifespan IQ change. By designing a study that was both longitudinal and cross-sectional he has shown that performance of older adults is maintained through the adult years with minimal decline occurring before age 60 to 70. However, each generation scores slightly higher on the IQ measures than the preceding one, and thus cross-generational comparisons disadvantage older cohorts. His conclusion is that each generation is slightly more intelligent than the preceding ones and that comparisons of 20-, 40-, and 60-year-olds show not declines in IQ scores but generational differences. Each generation maintains its scores, but succeeding generations score slightly higher, so that comparison makes it appear that decline has occurred. Persons who were initially tested when they were aged 25 or 32 have the highest scores. Those first tested at 39 or 46 have the next highest scores, and those who entered the testing situation at age 53, 60, or 67 have the lowest scores. However, scores for the youngest group show slight change over the 14-year period, scores for the middle group show no change at all, and scores for the oldest group decline substantially only after age 74. Schaie's data suggest clearly that intelligence as measured by the Thurstone Primary Mental Abilities Test is quite stable over the lifespan and that subsequent cohorts score better than preceding ones.

Age, of course, is not the only variable that affects IQ. Education, socioeconomic factors, and cohort are also major factors in determining the intelligence of any individual. Birren and Morrison[7] analyzed a large amount of data from the WAIS and concluded that education is much more important than age in determining the IQ of the individual. With increased education the IQ scores rise sharply. This does not necessarily mean that education increases IQ; it may mean that people with high IQ are prone to attend school longer or enjoy it more, or it may mean that there is some third factor involved that affects both IQ and education. Regardless of the causative relationship, increased education and higher IQ appear positively associated.

Likewise, greater socioeconomic status is associated with higher IQ scores. As noted earlier, crystallized intelligence is sensitive to experience and acquired information. These are likely to increase with higher socioeconomic status, since travel, a stimulating environment, availability of books, or encouragement of continued learning are more likely to be available for persons at a higher level of income, occupation, and education—the components of socioeconomic status.

We may conclude that intellectual potential is maintained throughout the major portion of the lifespan. *People even in their eighth decade have the ability to learn and change.* However, they often have not cultivated that ability and must expend additional energy to succeed in spite of the growing infirmities and difficulties. The role of the therapist is to understand the areas where additional help is needed and to design content and process so that learning can be maximized.

Implications

What implications may be drawn from studies of older adult intellectual performance? Regardless of their purpose, studies on intelligence in later life show clearly that in the verbal and sociocultural areas decline is least and comes latest. This suggests that the cognitive abilities of greatest relevance to the daily lives of older learners are those that evidence the most resistance to decline with age. Acquisition of knowledge or skill relevant to the older person's interests, needs, and wants should be learned quickly and efficiently. The *usefulness* of the content to the learner should be given special emphasis. If the topic is of interest and can be used in some important manner, the older person will be likely to learn.

Individual differences in intellectual performance (as well as practically every other variable) increase throughout the adult years. Thus in attempting to help older people learn the therapist must expect that the intellectual range will be great, experience will be diverse, and individual learning skills will differ extensively. The entire rehabilitation team must be flexible and work to individualize instruction.

LEARNING ABILITY AND PERFORMANCE IN LATER LIFE

Learning occurs throughout life. People continually learn through study, through incidental contact with others, through formalized contact with others (as a patient), through their jobs, and through analysis of their reactions and feelings. This learning process does not change abruptly when an individual reaches old age, but performance and ability differentials between older and younger people have been reported. This section emphasizes the measurement of learning performance and the means by which learning efficiency can be improved.

First, though, a caveat—learning and performance are not the same. Because an item has been learned does not necessarily mean that it can be recalled or recognized in every situation. In other words, poor performance on a learning task may mean that insufficient learning has occurred, or it may mean that the performance does not accurately reflect the extent of the learning achieved. However, it is only through the observation or measurement of performance that we can infer learning. Consequently, throughout this chapter, when learning is discussed it is the observable results of the learning that are measured and not some internal change that has taken place. Botwinick[3] has emphasized this distinction, and it should be kept in mind both in reviewing laboratory studies and in evaluating instruction of older people.

Over the past three decades a large number of laboratory studies of learning performance have provided extensive and reliable data on the changes that occur with age and that are especially amenable to intervention. The purpose of those studies has been to explore the age-related differences in learning performance (that is, the differences between older and younger learners). The review of these studies therefore will be selective in an attempt to abstract those of greatest relevance to the rehabilitation team. In so doing it is necessary to extrapolate from the findings in an attempt to suggest some instructional applications or principles. Thus our review of these studies attempts to provide a general understanding of the research, to report the more relevant findings, and to identify the implications and insights salient to persons attempting to help older people learn cognitive and/or motor skills.

Laboratory Study of Learning

Studies of learning performance have been conducted largely in a laboratory setting. Several experimental procedures have been used in which subjects either see or hear words, letters, or symbols and then are asked to recall or recognize them. In some studies paired words are presented, and the subject is expected to recall which word was matched with which other word. The specific design and method has varied widely, depending on the type of hypothesis being tested, but in general the subject attempts to memorize several words and to recall them after the passage of a short period of time.

Performance on learning tasks is affected by several factors. The intelligence of the individual, the learning skills acquired over the years, and the flexibility of learning styles are, of course, key variables. There are several other variables, however, often called noncognitive factors, that can also have a great effect on learning. These do not involve intellectual ability but nevertheless have a great bearing on the individual's performance. Noncognitive factors include the visual and auditory acuity of the learner, the health status of the individual, the motivation to learn, the level of anxiety, the speed at which the learning is paced, and the meaningfulness of the material to be learned.

Several of these are treated as major variables in research on learning performance; others, such as perceptual acuity and health status, in general are not. It should be obvious, however, that individuals who are unable to see or hear well are not likely to perform at an acceptable level. They will misunderstand directions, fail to adequately take in the material, and have a difficult time responding, particularly in written or oral form. These hindrances to learning do not relate to the individual's innate ability, but they interfere to such an extent that any learning performance is likely to be severely affected.

Likewise, poor health can be a major detriment in any learning situation. If the individual is not able to concentrate on the instruction because of pain, if physical stamina and strength are lacking, or if the senses are dulled through illness or medication, the learner will not be productive. Since the average number of days of illness per year increases with age, physical health of the individual must be considered in any measurement of learning performance and especially in any attempt to teach individuals or groups.

Thus attention to the noncognitive factors as well as the cognitive ones is important in designing a program of physical therapy and rehabilitation care that can induce the maximum physiologic capacity for patient participation.

Laboratory studies of learning in adulthood and later life have provided a wealth of data on the changes that occur in learning performance over the lifespan, the characteristics of this change, and the means by which learning performance can be improved in old age.

Interference.   Interference can cause a learning task to be less efficiently accomplished. Although Craik[8] argued that the data were inconclusive at best, most researchers seem to believe that interference can keep the individual from learning the new materials or substantially impede the learning process. There are several ways interference can occur. First, it can result from the conflict of present, personal knowledge with the new knowledge to be learned. Second, two learning tasks undertaken at the same time can interfere with each other. Third, subsequent learning can interfere with the intended learning. Each of these can prove to be a difficulty in the learning process.

Interference from prior events or knowledge has occurred in studies where older people were asked to learn nonsense words or symbols. On occasion, some of these symbols are contrary to common knowledge—for instance, "$6 + 2 = 3$." Arenberg and Robertson[9] report studies in which this type of learning proved to be substantially more difficult for older people than nonsense symbols that did not conflict with present knowledge (for instance, A + D = F). From a research point of view these equations are comparable; thus differences in the scores are attributed to conflict with present knowledge.

The rehabilitation team working with older people could utilize this understanding by emphasizing new knowledge that will be consistent with previous learning, by minimizing any conflicts between new and old knowledge, and by helping the older person unlearn incorrect knowledge. A specific implication of this understanding is that the practitioners can benefit from a familiarity with the older person and the beliefs, experiences, and knowledge he or she brings to the learning setting. If the new information is likely to be in sharp contrast with present knowledge, the therapist should proceed in a slow and careful manner, since overt or implicit resistance to the new information can be expected.

On the other hand, it is possible to use the past knowledge and experience of the older learner in a very positive and beneficial fashion. Studies have shown that older people benefit more than young adults when the material is familiar or consistent with what they already know.[9] The past experience and knowledge of the older person can be either positive or negative, depending upon its consistency or conflict with the new learning being undertaken, and it needs to be given special consideration by the therapist.

A second type of interference occurs when the older learner is expected to attend to two things at once. In laboratory studies this often occurs when subjects are expected to listen to different word lists in each ear simultaneously, remember which light was flashed a few seconds ago, or repeat words while listening to other words. In those studies where older people must divide their attention among intake, attention, and retrieval processes, they seem to be especially disadvantaged.[8, 9] When the older person is required to shift attention from one learning task to another, efficiency of learning suffers.

The implication of concurrent interference is that the therapist should concentrate on one task at a time and assure that one item is satisfactorily learned before the next is undertaken.[3] If a second task must be learned, it should be postponed as long as possible and should be clearly distinctive so that it is possible to know when one has completed the first task and is moving on to the next. Apparently, older people need more time to integrate the new learning and to rehearse it before it is well set in the secondary memory. Additional stimulation during this period is likely to result in premature forgetting or inability to adequately retrieve the information.

Another type of concurrent interference occurs from distractions at the time of learning. These may come from background noise, room conditions, personal anxiety, or numerous other factors. Whatever the cause, if the older individual divides attention betweeen the learning task and something else, learning speed and accuracy will decline. Thus the therapist is well advised to reduce the potential for distraction whenever possible and to help the older person concentrate exclusively on the learning at hand. This may not be easily done, but it is an effective means of increasing learning performance.

A third type of interference, retroactive interference, occurs when the individual completes one learning task and then must concentrate on some other task. This subsequent diversion may have a negative effect on retrieval of the first task, although this is not as well documented as are other types of interference.[10]

Therapists are advised to space the learning experiences of older people sufficiently to allow time for integration, to assure that the content does not conflict with previous learning, and to follow up at a later time to evaluate the quality of the knowledge retained. The possibility of retroactive interference is sufficient to encourage the therapist to incorporate review, reflection, and application of the learning.

Pacing.   Laboratory studies have shown that older people perform less well when the learning task must be completed under the pressure of time.[11, 12] Older people learn more successfully when they are provided additional time both to take in the information (presentation rate) and to retrieve the answer (response rate), although a slowed response rate appears to assist them most.[13] Paired associate tasks have proved especially difficult for older people, who do less well than younger people when tasks are to be completed quickly.[3] Canestrari[11] reported, however, that the learning deficiency can be somewhat overcome if the older learner is provided additional time and will almost disappear when the subject can control the learning pace. Thus when self-pacing by the older learner is allowed the learning performance appears to be optimized.[3, 14]

One implication of fast pacing in learning experiments is that older persons make more errors of omission, errors in which they make no response at all rather than risking a wrong answer. Omission errors are much more common to older learners and may result in part from inadequate time to determine the preferred response; therefore no response is made. Arenberg and Robertson-Tchabo[10] reported that additional time was useful in reducing the amount of nonresponse. When extra time is available it can lead to a successful search of secondary memory so that correct answers are forthcoming.

The application of this insight from laboratory research is very direct in a learning setting. Instruction should be self-paced or, if that is not possible, should be paced rather slowly in order to provide time for both intake and retrieval.[3, 14] Since a presentation (even to a single individual) is a form of timed instruction, it should be structured in such a manner that material is presented, reviewed, and examined. This may be effectively supplemented by an opportunity for questions and discussion that allows it to be related to previous knowledge, offers time for consideration of the material, and can reduce the psychologic pressure of speeded learning. Group therapy or treatment of two patients at a time lends itself well to application of these principles.

The importance of controlling the pacing of instruction cannot be overemphasized. The laboratory learning studies, research on adult intelligence, and practical experience clearly indicate the need for slowly paced or self-paced instruction for older people. This will typically require the therapist to reduce the amount of content to be presented and to offer greater clarity, specificity, and depth rather than cover a number of diverse topics. In posing questions to older persons, increased time needs to be allowed for response and greater care taken in framing the questions so that they are specific and directed. A greater emphasis needs to be placed on the design of forms that can be easily completed by patients. The older adult will fill out forms if given forms that are readable (large print if needed) and written in appropriate language (nonmedical) and given the necessary time to complete the form at a leisurely pace.

Organization of Material. Learning performance depends in part on whether or not the individual is able to retrieve what has been learned. Within the information-processing model of learning, retrieval is primarily dependent upon the manner in which the information is organized or "filed" in the brain. By organizing information into categories and sequences, or by using some type of visual or mnemonic device, the individual is generally able to increase the quality of retrieval.

This scheme has been shown to be especially applicable to older persons. Older adults typically do more poorly than younger adults on learning tasks; in an attempt to provide explanations for this finding, in addition to pacing and interference effects, the extent to which persons use some kind of organizing strategy has been studied.[15] Evidence is persuasive that older persons are less likely than others to spontaneously organize as a way to help memory.[3,10] When investigators have encouraged older people to categorize words to be learned, scores have improved; when the organizing strategy was provided by the researcher, scores improved significantly. This appears to be especially true for older people who have poor verbal skills; for highly verbal older people, the weaknesses in their organizing strategies are less pronounced, and improvement is minimal with this type of assistance.

Learning performance of older people can be improved by assisting them to organize the material in better ways and by encouraging alternatives to rote memorization. This can be done through the provision of "advance organizers," aids to help learners appropriately direct their attention. Many older learners have difficulty following the content because they cannot anticipate what will be taught and do not see the whole that is being presented. It is often helpful to provide an introductory overview in which the entire lesson is given in outline form. This provides an early opportunity to see the "map" that is being followed, an insight especially useful for older people.[3]

Advance organizers can also provide the bridge between what the older person already knows and what is intended to be learned in the present session. They can indicate the size, shape, extent, and orientation of the content to be covered so that dimensions can be appreciated in advance. Specific examples of advance organizers include an outline of the session; sets of notes to follow; initial summaries of the content; or lists of facts, concepts, or issues to be examined. These, of course, need not be provided in written form; however, when presentation in writing is the procedure, it does offer a guide that can be reviewed by the learner at any time (presuming that the individual can process written instructions; for evaluation strategies refer to Chapter 4).

A related aspect of this topic may be seen in studies in which older people are asked to reorganize the knowledge before responding. For instance, they are read a list of words or numbers and then asked to repeat them in reverse order. Studies have shown that older people do significantly poorer on this type of activity than younger persons,[8] since they must not only remember the material but reorganize it. Thus the older person faces not only the learning problem but the interference effects of two different processes.

There are clear implications from this finding for instruction of older people. If the content is presented in one way and the older person is expected to apply it some other way, the transition may cause difficulty. This would generally mean that older people should not be expected to acquire abstract information and to make the transition to practical application themselves. The instruction should be provided in the format that is to be used whenever possible. Most therapists are probably familiar with the situation in which the older person takes what is said too literally and is unable to generalize or apply the material to comparable settings. The reorganization process is not an easy one, and it is one that should be minimized whenever possible.

Another means of improving learning performance is through the use of mediators—that is, the association of the word or information to be learned with some other word, image, or story that can be remembered easily. As with other organizing strategies, older people are less likely than younger ones to consciously and regularly employ some type of mediator. Rather, they are likely to use rote memorization in order to remember the new information. Studies have shown that when older persons are assisted in using mediators, their scores improve. Some researchers have hypothesized that visual mediators (such as forming a picture of the word or information) are more effective in improving learning performance than verbal mediators. However, Canestrari[12] found little difference between visual and verbal mediators; both were helpful in improving the organization and remembering of the new information.

Mediators are useful in showing the relationships between facts that are known and those that are being learned. They can tie the new information to the old and help to show where the new knowledge fits in the individual's scheme of organizing information. Since older people are not likely to automatically employ these mediational devices, their learning efficiency can be improved by helping them form pictures, stories, analogies, or examples in order to make the tie and find the organizing variable. This can be done through encouragement of note-taking so that the individual will indicate the new information and where it fits with the old. It can also occur by helping the individual develop little stories or pictures that help recall specific information.

Although not particularly useful in many situations, the chaining of words or ideas is helpful in recalling lists. Each item of a list is related by a story or picture to the next. Thus when the first word is recalled it should be possible to recall the whole list by remembering the ties (pictures) to each succeeding word. Another method is to relate the words in a list to a numbered series of learned words. For instance, if you remember that one is "fun" and relate the first word to it, it can be remembered easier; if two stands for "shoe" and the second word is related to shoe by a small story, it too may be more easily recalled.

The implication from these data on the use of organization and mediative devices in learning is that the therapist needs to provide the time and opportunity for the learners to apply the new information, either in a mnemonic or nonsense way, or to relate it to previous knowledge. This provides not only the additional time identified earlier as necessary, but the possible reduction of interference with previous knowledge. By use of these strategies and devices it is possible to improve the quality of learning, even though the amount of content covered may need to be reduced because of the time involved in the application process.

Motivation. It is generally accepted that older people are less motivated when approaching a learning task than are younger people. Obviously a desire to succeed and a commitment to conscientiously address the task are important elements in successful learning performance. Since older people are known to have less general interest in learning, and since many of the tasks involved in the various studies have relatively little meaning or relevance to the older person, it has been assumed that older learners do less well because they are less motivated. Hulicka[16] reported that older persons refused to continue to attempt learning tasks that involved "such nonsense." This type of reaction has been reported by other researchers and has sometimes been interpreted as indicating low motivation.

One means of increasing motivation is to make the learning undertaken more meaningful to the individual learner. Calhoun and Gounard[14] reported that older people learned significantly more highly meaningful material than they did medium or low meaningful material. They concluded that understanding the needs and wants of the older learner and directing the content toward those meaningful areas will result in greater motivation as well as greater learning by older students.

Another approach to meaningfulness may be through the level of concreteness of the material. Several studies have pointed out the decline in abstract behavior with increased age;[3] older people may be unable or unwilling even in the laboratory to deal with problems distant from present reality. Arenberg[17] reported that when learning tasks were presented with abstract elements (forms, colors, numbers), older people had an extremely difficult time completing the tasks; however, when the elements were changed to more concrete items (specific beverages, meats, vegetables), the older learners accomplished the task much more easily. Thus it would appear advisable to present instructional components in ways as concrete as possible and as personally meaningful to the other student.

Other researchers have found contradictory results when measuring the motivation of older people in a learning task. Powell et al.[18] took blood samples and measured galvanic skin response and heart rate of older subjects involved in a learning study; they reported that older persons had higher levels of arousal—indicating greater involvement—than younger subjects. Older people experienced greater stress in the learning situation and performed the learning task more poorly than did younger persons.

Subsequent studies[19] have shown that if the degree of arousal is reduced by medication, the older learners improved their performance. This suggests that the older learner may be so motivated or involved in the study that emotional state interferes with the cognitive processes. By overreacting to the stress of the situation, the subject may withhold responses, score poorly on the learning task, and further increase anxiety in a vicious cycle.[20]

One means of overcoming this overarousal is by providing a supportive learning environment. If older people are placed in a situation in which they are expected to compete with others or be evaluated on their performance, they are likely to be overaroused and to do less well. Ross[21] reported a study in which three different sets of instructions were given to groups of older subjects; one set was considered to be supportive, one neutral, and one challenging. Older persons did best when given the supportive instructions, less well with neutral instructions, and least well with challenging instructions. The conclusion was drawn that positive expectation and supportive learning situation are likely to reduce the threat of the learning experience and to result in greater learning.

It has long been assumed that when correct responses are rewarded and incorrect ones are not, subjects will learn most quickly. A study by Leech and Witte[22] indicated that when all responses were rewarded—correct ones more strongly than incorrect ones—older persons could be persuaded to make some response to each question and thus reduce errors of omission. Learning tends to be poorer when the learner does not respond in some way; rewarding every response assists older persons to take a chance and perhaps learn something in that process.

The implications of these motivation studies are important, for the teaching of older adults. First, it should be obvious that older people will be more highly motivated if they are learning meaningful material. Their interest will be heightened, and their commitment is likely to be better. It is thus imperative that the relevance of the information presented be made clear and that its utilization be emphasized.

Second, if anxiety causes a decrease in learning efficiency, then the instruction should be carried out in a way that will reduce the fear of failure. This can occur primarily through the attitude and approach that the therapist brings to the learning setting. By presenting material at an appropriate level of complexity, by setting a relaxed pace, and by reducing the threat of failure, the therapist can make the learning experience more successful and enjoyable.

Third, the reward for participation in the learning setting should be clear and regular. To assume that the older person is able to stand defeat and has the necessary self-confidence to persevere regardless of the results may be inaccurate. The need for constant monitoring of the supportiveness of the climate, of the extent to which older people feel a part of the situation, and of the extent to which they are appreciated and valued regardless of their achievement is necessary for continued involvement and progress. Most important, however, is the clarity and meaningfulness of the learning undertaken. In order to maintain motivation the outcomes must be clear and closely related to the wants and interest of the older participants.

Sensory Modality.   Several studies have attempted to determine whether visual or auditory input is more effective in learning. Although all of us learn both by seeing (reading) material as well as by hearing (listening to) the spoken word, questions have been raised about the extent to which one is superior to the other. McGhie et al.[23] reported that auditory means are generally slightly superior to visual when the information is to be retrieved within a very short period of time. Visual means, on the other hand, may be superior if the information is to be held in the long-term memory for some period.[24]

Several studies have attempted to determine if learning is improved when one type of presentation (visual or verbal) is supplemented with the other. If the learner is provided visual images and hears the same material simultaneously, learning should be improved; in general this has proved to be the case.[17] Results of studies wherein subjects are present with one of three experimental conditions—looking at a list of words, looking at the words while the experimenter reads them (passive), or looking at the words and reading them aloud (active)—support the hypothesis that supplementation in either the active or passive form is valuable, with active supplementation the most helpful.

These studies suggest that therapists may facilitate learning by using both of the major senses, especially when this can be done simultaneously. When written material is provided for the learner to follow while a presentation is being made, increased learning is likely to result. However, there is a caution that must be added; if the verbal and the visual presentations are not similar, the older individual may experience interference from divided attention. Thus if the written materials are quite different from the verbal presentation, less rather than more learning may result. The therapist/teacher must carefully choose the material to be presented in written form so that it conforms closely to the presentation. Simply finding a seemingly relevant pamphlet or other handout may not be enough.

Another inference that may be drawn from the studies of modality relates to the active/passive aspect of the learning. Persons who were active in the learning process, even in such a minimal way as saying aloud the words to be learned, succeeded to a much greater extent. Most therapists have assumed that activity was a valued part of the learning enterprise, but this underscores the need to continue involvement of the older client, to seek ways for activity related to the new learning, and to encourage the older person to do more than attempt passively to "soak up" the knowledge.

Feedback.   Studies have shown that older persons are assisted in their learning when they are provided feedback on their performance.[25,26] Since the older individual often continues to use improper or ineffective means to address problem-solving or learning situations even after these have proved unproductive, the feedback is especially useful when it includes suggestions for alternative approaches.

The implications for instruction include the obvious value of allowing the older learner an opportunity to rehearse the behavior or learning under the guidance of the therapist so that corrective feedback can be provided. Since the older person typically requires a longer time period and a greater number of trials in order to achieve the desired learning, feedback on the amount of progress being made and the current level of functioning is generally of value.

As with most suggestions improperly applied, negative results can occur. Older people are typically less able to accept negative feedback and continue to do well. Since they often have less interest, greater anxiety, and lower self-concept, they are likely to experience greater detrimental results from negative feedback. Thus every attempt should be made to avoid a judgmental, critical position with a more supportive, helpful posture taken whenever possible.

Similarly, older people should be helped to avoid errors to the extent possible. Since they tend to remember errors and repeat them, it is most advisable to design the situation so that successful completion of the task is likely.[9] With mistakes, the self-concept of the older person is likely to fall, and continuing commitment to the learning experience will be reduced.

SUMMARY AND CONCLUSION

The central premise of this chapter is that older adults can and do learn effectively. Helping them to do so is both an art and a science; it will be most successfully accomplished when knowledge of intelligence, learning ability, and teaching techniques is combined with personal judgment characterized by flexibility and a positive attitude toward the learning potential of older persons.

The research reviewed in this chapter leads to several conclusions of relevance for the therapist working with older persons. First, while there are some aspects of intelligence that do indeed decline with age, other aspects appear to improve. On balance, intelligence typically remains fairly stable until late in life, and differences in intelligence among individuals are likely to be far more significant than differences in intelligence based merely on age.

Second, learning ability does not abruptly change in old age, but a modest decline in performance appears to occur, owing in part to noncognitive factors. Older persons requiring therapeutic intervention may experience at the outset even greater difficulty in learning because of such factors. Performance may be affected by depression, poor health, sense of loss of autonomy, or fear and unfamiliarity with the treatment setting, in addition to other noncognitive factors noted in this chapter.

Understanding such factors and their implications for the learning performance of older persons can help the therapist to modify this decline. Techniques suggested by these implications include minimizing the effects of interference from prior knowledge by basing new knowledge on old; allowing for self-pacing of instruction; facilitating the organization of materials; ensuring the relevance of materials presented; using both visual and verbal modes of instruction; and providing constructive feedback.

Despite changes in intelligence and learning performance, it is evident that older persons can learn and that well-planned instruction can facilitate learning efficiency and effectiveness. Understanding both the limitations and potentials of older adults and integrating that understanding with specific techniques will help therapists design quality instructional experiences for their clients.

The reader is referred to the work of Botwinick,[3] Knox,[2] Birren and Schaie,[27] and Jarvik et al.[28] for further study.

REFERENCES

1. Cattell RB: Theory of fluid and crystallized intelligence: A clinical experiment. J Educ Psychol 54:1–22, 1963.
2. Knox AB: Adult Development and Learning. Jossey-Bass, San Francisco, Calif., 1977.
3. Botwinick J: Aging and Behavior: A Comprehensive Integration of Research Findings. Springer Publishing Co., New York, 1978.
4. Eisdorfer C, Busse EW, Cohen LD: The WAIS performance of an aged sample: The relationship between verbal and performance IQs. J Gerontol, 14:197–201, 1959.
5. Riegel KF, Riegel RM: Development, drop, and death. Dev Psychol 6:306–319, 1972.
6. Schaie KW: Age changes in adult intelligence. In: eds. Woodruff DS, Birren JE Aging: Scientific Perspectives and Social Issues, Van Nostrand Reinhold, New York 1975.
7. Birren JE, Morrison DF: Analysis of the WAIS subtests in relation to age and education. J Gerontol 16:363–369, 1961.
8. Craik FIM: Age differences in human memory. In: eds. Birren JE, Schaie KW. Handbook of the Psychology of Aging, Van Nostrand Reinhold, New York, 1977.
9. Arenberg D, Robertson EA: The older individual as a learner. In: Education for the Aging, ed. Grabowski SM, Mason WD, ERIC Clearinghouse on Adult Education Syracuse, N.Y., n.d.
10. Arenberg D, Robertson-Tachabo EA: Learning and aging. In: eds. Birren JE, Schaie KW, Handbook of the Psychology of Aging, Van Nostrand Reinhold, New York 1977.
11. Canestrari RE, JR. Paced and self-paced learning in young and elderly adults. J Gerontol 18:165–168, 1963.
12. Canestrari RE, Jr: Age changes in acquisition. In: Human Aging and Behavior, ed Talland GA, Academic Press, New York, 1968.
13. Monge R, Hultsch D: Paired-associate learning as a function of adult age and the length of the anticipation and inspection intervals. J Gerontol 26:157–162, 1971.
14. Calhoun RO, Gounard BR: Meaningfulness, presentation rate, list length, and age in elderly adult's paired associate learning. Educ Gerontol 4:49–56, 1979.
15. Hultsch D: Adult age differences in the organization of free recall. Dev Psychol 1:673–678, 1969.
16. Hulicka IM: Age differences in retention as a function of interference. J Gerontol 22:180–184, 1967.
17. Arenberg D: Concept problem solving in young and old adults. J Gerontol 23:279–282 1968.
18. Powell AH Jr, Eisdorfer C, Bogdonoff MD: Physiologic response patterns observed in a learning task. Arch Gen Psychiatry, 10:192–195, 1964.
19. Eisdorfer C, Nowlin F, Wilke F: Improvement of learning in the aged by modification of autonomic nervous system activity. Science, 170:1327–1329, 1970.
20. Elias MF, Elias PK: Motivation and activity. In: Handbook of the Psychology of the Aging, eds. Birren JE, Schaie KW, Van Nostrand Reinhold, New York, 1977.
21. Ross E: Effect of challenging and supportive instructions in verbal learning in older persons. J Educ Psychol, 59:261–266, 1968.
22. Leech S, Witte KL: Paired-associate learning in elderly adults as related to pacing and incentive conditions. Dev Psychol, 5:180, 1971.
23. McGhie A, Chapman J, Lawson JS: Changes in immediate memory with age. Br J Psychol 56:69–75, 1965.

24. Taub HA: Mode of presentation, age, and short term memory. J Gerontol 30:56–59, 1975.
25. Hornblum JN, Overton WF: Area and volume conservation among the elderly: Assessment and training. Dev Psychol, 12:68–74, 1976.
26. Schultz NR, Hoyer WJ: Feedback effects on spatial egocentrism in old age. J Gerontol, 31:72–75, 1976.
27. Birren JE, Schaie KW (ed): The Handbook of the Psychology of Aging. Van Nostrand Reinhold, New York, 1977.
28. Jarvik LF, Eisdorfer C, Blum JE (eds): Intellectual Functioning in Adults. Springer Publishing Co., New York, 1973.

4 Psychosocial Dysfunction in the Aged: Assessment and Intervention

Kenneth Solomon

The elderly suffer from a greater incidence of psychopathology than any other age group. Over 50 percent of the elderly are at risk for developing a major psychopathologic dysfunction at some point in their life after age 65. The prevalence of psychopathology in the institutionalized elderly may be greater than 75 percent. Major physical illness with chronic limitation of function further increases the risk of the older person developing a psychopathologic disorder. The older person's mental status will have major ramifications for functional prognosis and response to physical therapy and rehabilitation.

Physical therapists are more likely than most other health professionals to spend a good portion of their professional time with the elderly population. Because physical therapists come into frequent contact with older people, accurate assessments become necessary for the appropriate treatment of the older patient. Being able to identify psychologic and social consequences of functional deficits and psychosocial factors that influence outcome will allow the physical therapist to function in a more productive and clinically successful manner. Most physical therapists know, for example, that the depressed patient is less likely to be motivated in physical therapy and is less likely to respond to interventions.

Knowledge of other stresses and resources in the psychosocial environment may make a world of difference in the outcome of treatment of the older person. For example, two men in their 80s suffered from severe functional disabilities, including apraxias, aphasias, and hemiparalyses, after a series of cerebrovascular accidents. One man was a childless widower whose only relative in the area was an older and frail sister. The other man had a devoted wife who was willing and capable of learning basic physical therapy skills. The first man was placed in a long-term-care institution following his discharge from the hospital. In spite of active rehabilitation and nursing interventions, he developed recurrent decubiti and secondary infections and died within 2 years after his stroke. The second man went home with his wife and received outpatient physical therapy. His wife made sure that he exercised daily, both actively and passively, and took care of his basic psychosocial and biologic needs. His family visited frequently, and with the help of some stronger family members he was able to be carried downstairs to a chair outdoors in the springtime. Although he suffered from several minor setbacks, this man stayed at home until his death in his sleep 7 years after discharge from the hospital.

Knowledge of psychogeriatrics also will help clear up misconceptions about and stereotypes of elderly patients that get in the way of appropriate treatment. Terms such as paranoia, depression, and acting out have become virtually meaningless jargon because usage of these terms has moved beyond their specific scientific meaning.[1] Other terms, such as senility or cerebral arteriosclerosis, have no place in the language of the health care professional, since these words are totally meaningless; indeed, they represent myths. Other words—e.g., manipulative—may be used for their pejorative connotation without the realization that its usage is a staff reaction to and labeling of certain disliked patients.[2]

This chapter presents an overview of psychogeriatrics. Issues and techniques of assessment of the elderly patient with psychosocial dysfunctions are discussed, and common psychopathologic syndromes that present in older people are reviewed. Principles and techniques for intervention are also discussed. Throughout the entire chapter the orientation is for the clinical physical therapist and members of the rehabilitation team, emphasizing the types of problems with which these health care providers come into contact.

NORMALITY AND PSYCHOPATHOLOGY

Normality, although a word used glibly every day, is virtually impossible to define. It has been used in many ways by a variety of clinicians with different approaches. The four major conceptualizations of normality used in health care, based on the work of Offer and Sabshin,[3] are presented here.

The first concept is normality as average. Normality used this way is based on statistics—mean, median, mode. For example, normal laboratory values for certain bodily components are expressed as a range derived from the mean plus or minus two standard deviations for the person's age and sex in that laboratory. Sociologically, this translates to behavioral norms, which are behaviors expected of an individual (actor) in a given role in a specific social situation based on expectations of behaviors that most people in such a setting would display.[4] However, judgments based on societal values bias the labeling of "statistical deviations" as pathology. For example, most people who are intelligent are statistically abnormal—their IQs are outside the range of two standard deviations—but are not considered pathologic. Similarly, people who behave in a societally deviant way are also abnormal because their behavior does not conform to the social norms; these individuals, however, are labeled "mentally ill."[5–7]

A second concept of normality is that of normality as utopia. It was embodied by Freud in his legendary statement that the goals of psychologic functioning are *lieben und arbeiten,* to love and to work. By this he meant that the psychologically "normal" adult is involved in a long-term, committed, one-to-one, intimate, heterosexual relationship and lifelong meaningful work, both conditions free of conflicts from previous stages of psychologic development. More recently, the "human potential movement" has translated this into self-knowledge and awareness of all one's conflicts, so that one can "work through" them and "grow" to a higher level of functioning; this process is called self-actualization.[8]

A third concept of normality is normality as the absence of disease. Using the broader World Health Organization definition, it would be the absence of dis-ease or physical, emotional, or social discomfort. This concept fits most acute medical or emotional dysfunctions but not other situations. For example, a person may repeatedly behave in a socially maladaptive way but not be uncomfortable. Although this behavior might be considered evidence of a personality disorder, it is also the absence of disease. Similarly, a patient with hypertension who is asymptomatic and totally unaware of the pathologic process in his or her body would be considered healthy by this concept. It also does not take into account a variety of common and not uncomfortable physical entities such as birthmarks (which are considered by dermatopathologists to be "abnormal").

The fourth concept of normality is normality as alloplasticity. Alloplasticity is the ability to manipulate both oneself and one's environment to meet one's needs and to manipulate one's needs to meet the needs of the environment. It includes the ability to actually create a new psychosocial environment if necessary. (In some ways this definition differentiates human beings from other forms of animal life.) Alloplasticity involves not only self-knowledge and growth but the development of skills of coping with an unpredictable biopsychosocial environment with subsequent flexibility and adaptability. In some ways it is related to normality as utopia, but it does not involve or demand the goal of conflict-free experience. On the contrary, it assumes that although many areas of ego functioning are conflict-free, human beings as complex animals can never be completely conflict-free but can learn to utilize the results of these conflicts to manipulate their environment and themselves to get their needs satisfied. This is an important concept for physical therapists, involving as it does the basic goals of rehabilitation.

Based on the alloplasticity concept of normality, psychopathology can be defined as follows: Psychopathology includes all forms of behavior [action, affect (or emotion), and cognition (or thought)] that interferes with or blocks an individual's alloplastic capabilities, causes discomfort for the individual and/or those around

that person, and is not a self-limited response to transitions and crises in the lif
cycle. It thus excludes responses to "problems of daily living" or adjustmen
disorders but includes most major disturbances as defined in the *Diagnostic an*
Statistical Manual, Third Edition[9] of the American Psychiatric Associatio
(DSM-III).

TYPES OF ASSESSMENT

There are four major types of psychosocial assessments of the elderly. Each fol
lows a different model. Each was developed by different disciplines, and eac
gives important information about the older person. The first three major types c
assessment are quite traditional in orientation and conceptualization. These ar
the diagnostic assessment, psychodynamic assessment, and the assessment c
needs. The fourth, the comprehensive psychogeriatric evaluation, is discusse
below. The information obtained by all four assessments overlaps to some degre
and the process of getting this information is identical for all four. They diffe
primarily in comprehensiveness of data collection and in how the data are orga
nized and translated into intervention.

The Diagnostic Assessment

The diagnostic assessment is based on the medical model. In it, objective sig
and subjective symptoms, along with other objective data, are combined under a
few labels as is necessary to explain the entire clinical picture (syndromes). F
example, a person who was previously in good health develops changes in level
consciousness over a period of several minutes, with symptoms of confusion an
anxiety, dizziness, and loss of motor power in one half of the body. Objective sig
include a hemiparesis, a hemianopsia, and a variety of other neurologic finding
Ancillary data would include increased uptake on a radioisotope brain scan, a
area of increased radiolucency on computerized axial tomography of the hea
and focal slowing on the electroencephalogram. A diagnosis can be made of
cerebrovascular accident, probably from an embolism.

In the psychosocial sphere, a similar diagnostic process leads the examiner
combine signs, symptoms, and other ancillary data in labels codified and define
in DSM-III. Familiarity with this work is necessary in communicating with ps
chiatrists and in order to understand the diagnostic shorthand and jargon er
bodied in DSM-III. It should be remembered that any diagnosis is just a label,
metaphor, to allow clinicians to communicate simply, a clinical shorthand used
that one does not have to list all the signs and symptoms of each patient ea
time.[10] It may also lead to specific biologic/medical interventions. For example,
diagnosis of a major depressive disorder is an indication for treatment with an
depressant medication and psychotherapy, while a diagnosis of an adjustment di
order with depressed mood is an indication for treatment with psychothera
alone.

The Psychodynamic Assessment

The psychodynamic assessment embodies another way of looking at a person's behavior, one derived from the work of psychologists. Rather than examining the end results of the psychologic problems as a medical syndrome with a diagnosis (e.g., depression or schizophrenia), the psychodynamic assessment attempts to evaluate some of the unconscious and interpersonal motivations for the person's behavior in an attempt to understand the roots of this behavior. It dictates psychologic/interpersonal interventions based on uncovering, clarifying, and gaining mastery over these unconscious and interpersonal motivations, with secondary change in behavior. Although psychoanalysis is the prototype of this modality, almost all psychotherapies, regardless of theoretical backbone, follow this model.

Assessment of Needs

A third model is derived from an assessment of needs. Based on the work of social workers, it conceptualizes the person from a functional point of view. It examines the needs that persons have and how well they are satisfying these needs. Maslow[8] has identified three types of needs: basic needs (food, water, touch, love), esteem needs (interpersonal interactions, caring, validation from others), and metaneeds (self-actualization).[9]

In some ways needs assessment is very simple. In physical therapy, for example, if a person with a need to be mobile suffers from a hemiparesis, this need is not being satisfied. The physical therapist has certain skills to help a person satisfy a given need, the satisfaction of which will also impact on the satisfaction of other needs (such as, in our example, the need to be autonomous and independent and the need to have a meaningful role). These become secondary issues to the immediate task at hand (improving mobility) although they have major psychosocial importance to the patient.

THE PSYCHOGERIATRIC EVALUATION

The fourth kind of assessment, and most comprehensive, is the psychogeriatric evaluation. As I see it, it is an attempt to gather and integrate biologic, psychologic, and social data so that a comprehensive understanding of the person's psychosocial state can be achieved. Problems are then delineated along a hierarchy of needs, and appropriate interventions are developed.

The psychogeriatric evaluation has 11 components. It is presented in its entirety in this chapter, but the physical therapist, as a member of the rehabilitation team, is neither expected nor required to be responsible for the entire evaluation. Many authors[11-20] have examined the roles of various mental health professionals and have divided them into two major categories: generalist and specialist roles. Generalist roles are those clinical roles not limited by disciplinary boundaries or training. Rather, these roles are used by all professionals in the fulfillment of various professional tasks. They are discussed in more depth elsewhere.[11-12, 18-20] Specialist roles differentiate among different professionals on the team and utilize specific skills, knowledge, and personality traits of these professionals in the total care of the individual.

Most work accomplished in the psychosocial aspects of caring for the elderly person in a rehabilitation setting utilizes generalist skills of all members of the rehabilitation team. The psychogeriatric evaluation is one task that can be completed using only generalist skills. Thus physical therapists should be able to complete a psychogeriatric evaluation, if necessary, and be able to utilize that information to formulate a treatment plan that maximizes the rehabilitation potential of the individual. Physical therapists should be able to understand the work of other professionals on the team so as to be able to interact professionally and communicate effectively, thus maximizing team functioning.[21-23] This procedure does not minimize the specialist roles of the physical therapist, roles that involve the various techniques used in physical therapy and rehabilitation.

The components of the psychogeriatric evaluation are discussed in turn.

History of the Present Episode

One needs to know exactly what the person is feeling and experiencing, how long it has been going on, what seemed to trigger it, what makes it better (even temporarily), what seems to make it worse, and what interventions the patient and family and mental health personnel have tried hoping to improve this particular problem. It is in the history of the present episode that one asks the specific questions regarding the various symptoms—including presence or absence of vegetative, depressive, psychotic, phobic, and obsessive-compulsive symptoms—needed to make a diagnosis as well as to assess blocks in need satisfaction.

Past Psychiatric History

One not only needs to ask if the person has had inpatient or outpatient psychiatric treatment in the past, but whether or not the person has received intervention for emotional problems from other personnel, such as psychologists, social workers, psychiatric nurses, and clergy. In addition, knowledge of any history of receiving "nerve pills" or other psychotropic drugs from a family physician is important. This information will help clarify a person's ability to cope and the coping mechanisms. The presence of a history of a severe psychiatric disability would be an indication either for a prescription of specific interventions (especially psychopharmacologic) that have been successful in the past[24] and the avoidance of interventions that have been previously proved unsuccessful.

Past and Present Medical Status

Knowledge of the person's medical history is necessary to assess the person's overall functional capabilities and to know what problems to expect in the future. The presence or absence of certain medications may impair or enhance the overall rehabilitation process. This history may also hint at certain somatic disorders or medications that may be causing the psychopathology noted (e.g., depression secondary to hypothyroidism or toxic psychosis secondary to antidepressants).

Drug History

The patient's use of drugs must be ascertained, including not only prescription medications but also over-the-counter drugs and street drugs. Many older people have problems with alcohol or drugs that may interfere with the patient's overall functioning as well as with the rehabilitation program or may otherwise cause specific psychiatric disorders. Besides alcohol, the most commonly abused drugs in the elderly are over-the-counter "nerve pills," benzodiazepines, marijuana, barbiturates, amphetamines, and legal narcotic analgesics; any use of these drugs must be specifically ascertained.

Psychosocial Evaluation

The purpose of the psychosocial evaluation is to gather information about the person's past coping skills and about factors that may enhance or inhibit psychiatric and physical rehabilitation, and to assess other stresses and resources in the patient's environment.

The psychosocial evaluation begins with a family history, including information about the patient's parents, siblings, and children. It also includes the medical and psychiatric history of these individuals and what kind of relationships these people had and have with each other and with the patient. In addition, the family history includes occupational and social class background of the patient's parents (and whether or not they were immigrants) and the relationship between the parents.

In the developmental history, the person's meeting of developmental landmarks is assessed. The examiner also gathers information about the person's childhood.

In the educational history, one asks questions about the person's level of education and use of this education. Why a person stopped or continued educational pursuits at different times is ascertained and interest in lifelong learning, vocational rehabilitation, and attitude toward education are assessed.

In the person's occupational history the examiner looks at jobs held, ability to hold a job, and the kind of work the person is interested in. One also examines for exposure to occupational hazards that might have diagnostic or therapeutic implications.

In the marital and sexual history one examines these relationships as a major resource and/or stress regardless of marital status, sexual orientation, or sexual exclusivity or nonexclusivity. If the patient has never married or cohabited with someone, the reasons for this need to be assessed. The entire spectrum of the individual's interpersonal relationships is examined in this way. One also ascertains the patient's interest in and level of sexual activity, with its obvious implications for rehabilitation.

One then looks at the person's current financial situation. This includes examination not only of sources of income but includes other social services that substitute for income—e.g., health insurance coverage and nutrition programs.

The examiner then investigates the patient's current housing for the presence and absence of barriers and to see how the house can be made barrier-free. Thus housing can be both a stress and a resource to the individual.

How the person uses leisure time is also assessed. This assessment is important not only in planning relaxation for the patient but also to gather information about the patient's ability to relax, experience positive affects, and develop meaningful rather than just time-consuming activities.

In planning a rehabilitation program as well as psychotherapy, knowledge of the person's premorbid personality is crucial. This information will tell the therapist what kind of defenses and coping mechanisms the person uses. The examiner will also learn how the person has satisfied various needs in the past and whether or not the person has been capable of adapting to stress in the past. This information will clarify other psychologic stresses and resources the individual brings into the rehabilitation situation and will help to assess the risk of the individual developing major psychopathology in the future. For example, people with labile personality disorders are at risk for developing depression, and those with stable personality disorders are at risk for developing either depression or paraphrenia when stressed in old age.[25-27] People without personality disorders are more likely to cope successfully with stress. At the same time that one assesses the premorbid personality of the patient, one examines the entire environment to assess other stresses and resources present.

Review of Systems

While such review has traditionally been part of the medical examination, it can be done by any health professional. The examiner asks about various symptoms of disease, including pain, visual problems, bowel habits, diet and appetite, sleep, and sexual functioning. Formal guides to a review of systems have been published elsewhere.[28-31]

Physical Examination

The physical examination should be complete, including rectal and pelvic examination. Although this must be done by a physician, nurse practitioner, or physician's assistant, the physical therapist must be apprised of this information in order to understand the problems of the older person and plan appropriate interventions.

Neurologic Examination

Since many older individuals in the rehabilitation setting have or are suspected to have neurologic disease, a thorough neurologic examination must be done. This does not have to be done by a neurologic consultant, since all physicians and other health professionals who do physical examinations are trained to perform neurologic examinations. The information garnered must be transmitted to the members of the rehabilitation team.

Mental Status Examination

There are 15 parts of the mental status examination. Part of the mental status examination involves observation of the patient during the conduct of the psychogeriatric examination rather than as a separate part of the formal examination.

Delineation of psychopathologic symptoms is necessary for an accurate assessment of the psychosocial status of the older patient. Accurate, value-free descriptions of behavior, without labels, are the backbone of the mental status examination. In reviewing the mental status examination, one can easily see many forms of behavior varying from the expected normative behavior of the patient. These variations are not necessarily psychopathologic. For example, a sad affect would be very appropriate to someone who has recently had a cerebrovascular accident but would not be appropriate for someone who has just won a lottery. There are several descriptions of the conduct of the mental status examination.[32-34]

Appearance. First, one notes the patient's appearance. How is he or she dressed? Is she or he in a bed or wheelchair, or ambulatory? What is his or her posture? Are there any other signs that might indicate the possibility of physical disease? Appearance is either appropriate or inappropriate for the patient's medical condition and social setting. For example, it generally would not be considered appropriate for a patient to wear pajamas to an outpatient appointment, but it is appropriate to wear them in a hospital. The social context of a patient's appearance must be taken into account. The same holds true for posture, which may be relaxed, tense, indicative of physical pathology, or bizarre and unusual as in some psychotic individuals.

Level of Consciousness. One then notes the patient's level of consciousness and alertness. The level of consciousness may be normal, or the patient may be hyperalert with wide eyes, scanning the environment. The patient may be hypoalert or may be drowsy, sleeping, obtunded, semicomatose, or comatose.

Attention Span. The third part of the examination is evaluation of the patient's attention span. The patient may have marked difficulty paying attention because of distractibility or hearing deficit. On the other hand, a patient may be demonstrating denial or selective inattention or may for unconscious reasons not attend to the examiner. Selective inattention is usually under some conscious control, but denial is not. Distractibility is usually noted in those with severe psychotic or cognitive disorders.

Mood. Mood is ascertained by asking the patient how she or he feels and what the underlying mood is. For example, is the patient happy, sad, or angry? Mood may be happy or sad within the realm of human experience, or the patient may experience extremes of mood, including elation or euphoria on the one hand or severe depression on the other. The person may be angry or hostile or experiencing anxiety or fear.

Affect.   Associated with mood is the fifth parameter of the mental status examination, affect. This is the behavioral manifestation of the underlying mood, and it is usually ascertained through examination of the patient's facial expressions. Is the facial expression angry, sad, happy, dull, or blunted? Also, the examiner wants to know if the affect corresponds to the expressed thought content. The patient's affect may be appropriate or inappropriate. Inappropriate affect is affect that does not fit the underlying mood or the content of the person's thoughts. If inappropriate, it may also be blunted or flattened, which is when the person does not facially express underlying feelings.

Level of Activity.   Sixth, one examines the level of activity. Is it normally active, hyperactive, or hypoactive? Are there tremors or other abnormal movements? The patient may demonstrate psychomotor retardation, in which all physical functions are slowed up, or psychomotor agitation, in which there is restlessness or agitation. Mild agitation may be manifested by mild finger-tapping and hand-wringing. Severe agitation is manifested by a person having difficulty staying still for more than a few moments. This condition must be differentiated from akathisia, which is a common parkinsonian symptom.

Speech.   One then examines the quality of the patient's speech. One looks at the quantity, volume, tone, inflection, speed, and understandability (coherence) of speech. Speech may be incoherent or indistinct on the basis of aphasia or dysarthria. It may be rapid or slow, monotonous in tone and inflection, or too low or loud volume. It may or may not be appropriate to the situation, content, or affect.

Thought Processes.   The examiner then considers the patient's thought process. Is it rational, logical, and oriented toward a goal? Does the patient attempt to answer questions in a reasonably concise manner? Is the patient able to express thoughts clearly, or is there evidence of receptive and/or expressive aphasia? Deficiencies of thought include paucity of thought, which is a relative lack of expressed thought. Perseveration occurs when the same thought is expressed over and over again regardless of its relevance to the question asked. Other disorders of thought process include a loss of the normal logical pathways of human thought. When mild, this is called tangentiality, in which the person seems to constantly digress from the topic, or circumstantiality, in which the person "beats around the bush" but eventually answers the question. More severe loss of logical aspects of thought is called loose association or derailment. When severe, the person's speech may be almost impossible to understand. This situation is called a word salad. In addition, the patient may use neologisms, invented words that may have idiosyncratic meanings known only to the patient.

Thought Content.   Next, one examines the content of the patient's thought. What is the patient specifically thinking, and is it relevant to the business at hand? Disturbances of thought content are several. One is vagueness of thought. Other disturbances of thought include compulsive repetition or obsessive intrusion of a thought alien to the patient's ego. The person may demonstrate *idées fixes,* which are unshakable and encapsulated ideas that may or may not be delusional. The patient may also be preoccupied with phobic ideas or fantasies. The patient may demonstrate delusions, which may be reasonably logical beliefs that are not based in reality. Delusions are frequently paranoid in the elderly. They may be encapsulated or limited to only a small part of the patient's life and may not affect the patient's functioning in other ways, or they may be unencapsulated, global, and severely disruptive. They may be organized into a delusional system, or they may be disorganized. The patient may also demonstrate confabulation or may create "factual" information to cover up memory deficits; this must be differentiated from willful lying. Depressive thought content, including self-deprecation, statements of irrational guilt, and feelings of helplessness, hopelessness, worthlessness, and uselessness, may also be demonstrated.

Finally, certain specific Schneiderian first-rank symptoms of schizophrenia are included as disturbances of thought. These include thought insertion (the belief that an outside force or person is putting thoughts in a person's head), thought control (the belief that an outside force is controlling a person's thoughts), behavioral control (a similar belief associated with behavior), thought withdrawal (the belief that an outside force is taking thoughts out of a person's head), and thought broadcasting (the belief that people are able to hear the individual's thoughts out loud). Schneiderian first-rank symptoms are believed to be pathognomonic of schizophrenia in younger people[35] but have no specific pathognomonic consequence in the elderly.

Perception. In examining perception one is examining the person's ability to understand the spoken and written word as well as looking for unusual perceptual experiences. Many major disorders of perception are pathophysiologic in nature, including receptive aphasias and the results of major sensory deficits.

Another common disorder of perception is illusion in which things may be perceived in a manner different from a measurable reality. The optical illusion is one example with which most people are familiar. Misperceptions are another form of perceptual disorder, one in which something is misidentified as something that it is not. The most severe perceptual disorders are hallucinations, in which the person creates sensory inputs not based in the external environment; they may be auditory, visual, olfactory, gustatory, tactile, or kinesthetic. Specific Schneiderian perceptual symptoms include hallucination of two voices communicating with each other or hallucination of a voice keeping up a running commentary on the person's behavior.

Memory. Memory is examined, in part, during the process of obtaining a history, a process that allows the examiner to ascertain the accuracy of the patient's recent and remote memory. Questions about the patient's activities over the few days prior to the examination also tests recent memory. To test for immediate recall, one can give the patient three items to remember and check back several minutes later to see if they are recalled (but see also Chapter 5). Memory disturbances include specific amnesias and hypomnesias, as well as more global disturbances of immediate recall, recent memory, and remote memory and the part processes of registration, retention, recognition, and recall.

Orientation. One next tests for orientation. Does the patient know the day of the week, date, month, year, and season? Does the patient know the name of the place he or she is in, the address, the floor, the room number? Can the patient give a reasonable account of herself or himself? Is the patient aware of the present situation? (In other words, does the patient understand the environmental parameters surrounding him or her?) Difficulty with orientation is called disorientation; it is the person's inability to identify the time, the place, or basic information about herself or himself.

Intelligence.   One assesses the patient's level of intelligence by examining ability to perform higher cortical functions. Can the patient serially subtract seven from a hundred? Can the patient follow simple instructions? Can he or she read and write a simple sentence? How well does she interpret proverbial statements? Are the proverbs interpreted abstractly or concretely? The adages I usually use are "you can lead a horse to water but you can't make it drink" and "people in glass houses shouldn't throw stones." Can the patient identify similarities and differences between items such as an apple and an orange? Disorders of intelligence may include lifelong intellectual deficits, as in mentally retarded individuals, or acquired intellectual deficits. The latter may be specific, as dyslexia, or global, as in dementia, and may include difficulties following simple instructions, reading, calculating, and writing sentences. The deficit may also include loss of the ability to abstract proverbs, which is partially dependent upon both the educational level and cultural background of the patient.

Judgment.   One tests judgment by assessing what the patient would do in hypothetical situations. The situations I use are the following: "What would you do if you found a letter lying on the ground in front of a mailbox?" "What would you do if you smelled smoke while at the movies?" Responses give the examiner information about the patient's ability to integrate environmental cues and choose between several alternative behaviors. Difficulties of judgment include impulsivity, failure to take the consequences of one's behavior into account prior to action.

Insight.   The final part of the mental status examination is the assessment of the patient's level of insight. One asks the patient why she or he feels that the specific emotional, behavioral, or cognitive difficulty has developed. Levels of insight range from a complete denial of all symptoms, through the ability to identify symptoms but not consequences or etiology, through the identification of symptoms and consequences but not their etiology, to insight into the nature and cause of one's psychosocial difficulties. The level of insight will often dictate the type of intervention planned with the patient.

Laboratory Examination

The specific laboratory examination is dependent upon the nature of the psychologic difficulty considered. All geriatric patients who develop psychopathology should have a complete blood count, renal, liver, and thyroid function studies, electrolytes, fasting blood sugar, electrocardiogram, chest x-ray, serology for syphilis, and serum concentrations of drugs that the patient is taking. In addition, if a diagnosis of brain failure is being considered, the patient should also have vitamin B_{12} and folate blood levels assessed, along with an electroencephalogram and computerized axial tomography of the head. Other specific laboratory evaluations may also be necessary.

Social Examination

The social examination is the final part of the psychogeriatric evaluation. One includes information gathered from review of the patient's chart and discussions with social service staff, nursing staff, family members, neighbors, and other important individuals in the patient's life. It will corroborate the history the patient gives the examiner and also gives the examiner insight into other symptoms that the patient may be unwilling or unable to discuss with the examiner. It will also help assess and enlist the interpersonal resources available to the patient. If feasible, the social examination includes a tour of the patient's home to assess resources, stresses, and barriers in the environment.

INTERVIEWING TECHNIQUES

The psychogeriatric evaluation is not necessarily done in a rigid sequence such as that listed above. A specific rhythm develops in a good interview: First, one starts with very broad questions that avoid "yes" and "no" answers; gradually, more specific questions are asked. Then one returns to broad questions as new areas are explored. The entire evaluation takes 1 to 2 hours.

I usually start by first introducing myself to the patient, asking if I can sit on the bed or chair, and then asking the patient how he or she feels and also what it is that bothers her or him. The patient should always be given the opportunity to discuss the immediate problem and what is of utmost concern to him or her. The patient is allowed to discuss this at her or his own pace and rhythm. Specific questions are geared to clarifying particular points and filling in some gaps as they develop.

Once the history of the present episode is elicited, I then seek answers to specific items of the psychogeriatric examination, again beginning with broad questions. For example, I might ask something about what it was like growing up as a child. From there, I can ask more specific questions about parents, siblings, and other childhood experiences; gradually the entire evaluation is completed.

The interview should be private and confidential and conducted without the presence of friends, relatives, or other staff. As part of the social examination, however, these collateral individuals should be interviewed with the patient present, as keeping secrets from the patient is likely to cause strain in the therapist-patient relationship.

The examiner should strive for a friendly, frank, and outspoken relationship, since his or her own insecurity and anxiety will become apparent to the patient and interfere with the examination. In part this anxiety can be overcome by being clear in one's own mind about what facts are to be elucidated and how to approach the patient. As noted above, it is usually best to discuss some aspect of the present difficulty or primary complaint first and then proceed as naturally as possible to other parts of the examination. "Yes/no" questions and leading questions must be avoided at all times. Tact, gentleness, and respect for the patient's sensitivities are most essential. If the patient should suffer from a catastrophic reaction

Table 4-1. Mini-Mental State Examination

BEGIN HERE: Now I would like to ask you some questions to check your concentration and memory. Most of them will be easy.

What is the . . . *(RECORD ANSWERS AND CIRCLE APPROPRIATE CODE)*

		Correct	Error	Refusal Can't Do	Refusal Other Refusal
1.	. . . year?	1	2	6	7
2.	. . . season?	1	2	6	7
3.	. . . date?	1	2	6	7
4.	. . . day of week?	1	2	6	9
5.	. . . month?	1	2	6	7
6.	. . . Can you tell me where we are right now? For instance, what state are we in?	1	2	6	7
7.	. . . What city are we in?	1	2	6	9
8.	. . . What hospital are we in?	1	2	6	7
9.	. . . What building are we in?	1	2	6	7
10.	. . . What floor of the building are we on?	1	2	6	7

11–13. I am going to name three things. After I have said them, I want you to repeat them. Remember what they are because I am going to ask you to to name them again in a few minutes.

	Correct	Error	Can't Do	Other Refusal
Apple:	1	2	6	7
Table:	1	2	6	7
Penny:	1	2	6	7

Please repeat the three items for me.
"Apple" . . .
"Table" . . .
"Penny" . . .

SCORE FIRST TRY. REPEAT OBJECTS UNTIL ALL ARE LEARNED.

14–18. Can you subtract (take away) 7 from 100, and then subtract 7 from the answer you get and keep subtracting 7 until I tell you to stop?

Record ___ ___ ___ ___ ___
       (93) (86) (79) (72) (65)

Number of Errors: 0   1   2   3   4   5

Refusal: Can't do   6
          Other refusal   7

19–23. *ALTERNATIVE TO Q. 14–18.*
Now I am going to spell a word forward and I want you to spell it backward. The word is W-O-R-L-D. Spell "world" backward.

REPEAT IF NECESSARY, BUT NOT AFTER SPELLING STARTS.

Print Letter: ___ ___ ___ ___ ___

Number of Errors: 0   1   2   3   4   5

Refusal: Can't Do   6
          Other Refusal   7

24–26. Now what were the three objects I asked you to remember?

	Correct	Error	Refusal Can't Do	Refusal Other Refusal
Apple:	1	2	6	7
Table:	1	2	6	7
Penny:	1	2	6	7

		Correct	Error	Can't Do	Other Refusal
27.	*SHOW WRISTWATCH.* What is this called?	1	2	6	7
28.	*SHOW PENCIL.* What is this called?	1	2	6	7
29.	I'd like you to repeat a phrase after me:	1	2	6	7

"No ifs, ands, or buts."

ALLOW ONLY ONE TRIAL.

		Correct	Error	Can't Do	Other Refusal
30.	Read the words on this page and then do what it says.	1	2	6	7

CODE 1 IF PATIENT CLOSES EYES.

CLOSE YOUR EYES

Table 4-1. Continued

31–33.	*READ FULL STATEMENT AND THEN HAND OVER PAPER.*				
	I'm going to give you a piece of paper. When I do, take the piece of paper in your right hand, fold the paper in half with both hands, and put the paper down on your lap.	Right hand:	1	2	6	7
		Folds:	1	2	6	7
		In lap:	1	2	6	7
34.	Write a complete sentence on this paper for me.					
35.	Here is a drawing. Please copy the drawing on this page.					

SCORING FOR 34/35.

34.	*SENTENCE SHOULD HAVE A SUBJECT AND VERB AND MAKE SENSE. SPELLING AND GRAMMAR ERRORS ARE OKAY.*	1	2	6	7
35.	*CORRECT IF THE TWO FIVE-SIDED FORMS INTERSECT TO FORM A FOUR-SIDED FIGURE AND IF ALL ANGLES IN THE FIVE-SIDED FIGURE ARE PRESERVED.*	1	2	6	7

or become severely agitated, it is usually wise to terminate the interview and return at a future time. Note-taking interferes with observation and also is frequently objected to by many patients; therefore I suggest that any notes needed should be written immediately after the interview, when the therapist is alone.

One way of assessing many aspects of the patient's mental status, especially memory, orientation, and higher cortical functioning, is to use the Mini-Mental State Examination[36] (Table 4-1). The Mini-Mental State Examination has the advantage of being reproducible, quantitative, and quick (it takes less than 4 minutes to complete with the average patient). It gives important clues to possible deficits of higher cortical functioning.

Following completion of the interview, I always ask the patient if there is anything important that has not been touched upon that the patient wishes to share. I also tell the patient what I think about the patient's condition and what my plans are, even if my plans at that point are only to discuss the situation with the other members of the treatment team. I always give the patient the opportunity to question me, though I tactfully refuse to answer personal questions; instead, I limit questions to the clinical task. My interview is terminated with a request to see the patient again, with the patient's permission.

BLOCKS TO ADEQUATE ASSESSMENT

There are several factors that lead to an inadequate psychogeriatric assessment of elderly patients. Some of these blocks are based in the physical therapist's acceptance of societal attitudes toward and stereotyping of the elderly; others are an integral part of the structure of the delivery of health care services. Still others may be personal issues for the therapist, and others derive from the personality of the patient.

It is well known that health workers, regardless of specific profession, stereotype the elderly in exactly the same manner that the general population does (see various references cited in Refs. 22, 23, 25, and 37–41). Although there are no data specifically assessing the adherence of physical therapists to the stereotype, the consistency of data from other health professionals makes it reasonable to extrapolate such data to physical therapists.

Stereotyping has been defined by Solomon and Vickers[42] as "the holding in common of a standardized mental picture representing an oversimplified and uncritical judgment of another group." Stereotyping has been hypothesized to lead to the delivery of inadequate or inappropriate services to the elderly[43] (disputed by O'Dowd and Zofnass[44]) and is a factor in the development of learned helplessness in older people.[38,45,46] The stereotype of the elderly is as follows:[47]

1. They are conservative and old-fashioned.
2. They have limited activities and interests.
3. Physical deterioration is inevitable.
4. They are poor.
5. They have only negative or only positive personality traits.
6. They are dirty.
7. Mental deterioration is inevitable.
8. They interfere in the lives of others.
9. They are repudiated by their families.
10. They are asexual.
11. They are either in the best or the worst period of life.
12. They are pessimistic.
13. They are insecure and helpless.

As with all stereotypes, each of those statements is untrue for the elderly as a group, although some may be true for some older individuals.

By believing in this stereotype of older people, the health professional is likely to prelabel behaviors and feelings of the older patient, which may then lead to an inadequate and inappropriate diagnosis of "senility" or a belief that psychotherapeutic and sociotherapeutic modalities are not efficacious in older people. In addition, the health worker who believes in the stereotype is likely to design an environment and therapeutic culture that further reinforces the stereotype. These beliefs will also lead to an independence of response-outcome in interactions between the elderly patient and the therapist, thus leading to the development of learned helplessness.[38,45,46]

The second block to adequate assessment is ageism. Ageism is more than just discrimination on the basis of age; rather, it is an entire melange of negative societal attitudes and behaviors toward older people.[43] It encompasses the behavioral results of the stereotype described above but also includes four types of victimization (physical, economic, role, and attitudinal)[41,48] and resultant prejudice and misconceptions.

One type of medical model, the diagnosis-treatment model,[49] can be another factor that interferes with adequate assessment of older people. Negative attitudes and stereotypes will prevent even the use of this model, as they will preclude the accurate diagnosis of older people because of labeling. In addition, the medical problems of the elderly are almost always multiproblematic and not purely biologic. The use of this rigid model is in conflict with a systems model more appropriate to the medical care of the elderly, and its use is further complicated by the fact that common diseases may present in uncommon ways in older people.[50]

There is a second medical model, the organizational model, in which the physician is atop a pyramid of other health workers, giving orders and making all major decisions.[49] This model frequently leads to a narrow view of the older person and inadequate examination of factors that influence rehabilitation. It also leads to rigid role definitions, which have consequences for the functioning of the different team members.[19-20]

Besides stereotyping and ageism, there may exist unresolved personality issues for the therapist that may cause problems for assessment.[25,51] The therapist may either infantilize or parentify the older patient and be blind to these specific intergenerational issues that may affect therapy. The therapist may also avoid certain specific issues, especially sexuality, chronicity, and mortality, during the assessment or intervention process.

The patient may have difficulty responding to the assessment process. Patients with dysarthria and aphasias present particular problems, as do those with severe cognitive impairment and those demonstrating catastrophic reactions. Severely depressed people may also be difficult to evaluate, as are those who are actively psychotic. Yet it is imperative to do as complete an assessment of these individuals as possible. For example, severe depression may mimic dementia or aphasia; however, since depression is much more treatable than these other conditions, an accurate assessment is essential. Other psychologic issues in the patient may lead to blocks in assessment. The patient may infantilize or parentify the therapist[25,51] or refuse to deal with issues that are emotionally charged and laden with conflict, perhaps for an entire lifetime.

ASSESSMENT OF NEEDS

When the assessment data are collected, there is a need to organize them into a clinically useful paradigm. One such paradigm, developed by Vickers[52] and based on the work of Maslow,[8] allows for the development of a hierarchy of needs. The following discussion includes my minor modifications of Vickers' paradigm.

Maslow hypothesized that basic needs must be satisfied before one can successfully work toward the satisfaction of needs higher up the hierarchy. Blocks in satisfaction of these basic needs thus have implications for all needs of the hierarchical pyramid.

At the base of the pyramid are biologic needs. These are needs for physiologic homeostasis and absence of disease, including thirst, hunger, warmth, and other physical comforts. Problems that arise in this area are most commonly defined as medical problems. Problems may also include such biologically autonomous behaviors as panic and vegetative symptoms of depression. Biologically autonomous behaviors have physiologic concomitants and are self-perpetuating. Problems in this realm are treated by biologic methods, especially medication and surgery.

The next level of the pyramid includes activities of daily living. These are the skills that allow daily survival, including ability to find an adequate diet, pay one's bills, get adequate income, dress oneself appropriately for the weather, and self-advocacy. It is at this level that the physical therapist is most active, as much of rehabilitation involves the correction of or adaptation to blocks to a person's ability to manage activities of daily living. For example, physical therapists do not work with cerebrovascular accidents per se; rather, they deal with the functional sequelae of this biologic disorder. All blocks in activities of daily living, either physical or emotional, are treated with various rehabilitative and reeducative techniques.

On the third level of the hierarchy are social needs. These are needs to interact with others, to maintain meaningful social roles, and to avoid loneliness.[53] Problems in this realm may come from the individual because of inadequate social skills, social anxieties, or maladaptive interpersonal behaviors, or from society, including rigidly defined social and gender roles. Intervention at this level includes all therapies that involve the patient, the therapist, and at least one other person. Examples would include marriage counseling, group psychotherapy, and consciousness-raising groups.

These first three levels of needs are roughly equivalent to Maslow's basic needs. The next level of the hierarchy corresponds to Maslow's concept of esteem needs. This is the psychologic realm and includes such constructs as mood, affect, identity, self-esteem, and body image, as well as the need for love, validation, and security. These psychologic needs are primarily internal to the individual, although they may have interpersonal ramifications. Problems in the psychologic realm are handled through a variety of individual psychotherapies involving only the patient and the therapist, including psychoanalysis, psychoanalytic psychotherapy, supportive psychotherapy, transactional analysis, and Gestalt psychotherapy.

The peak of the pyramid corresponds to Maslow's metaneeds. These are creative and self-actualization needs, including the need to express oneself in a meaningful way along with various existential issues, such as the meaning of life, mortality, life goals, and one's *Weltanschauung*. The problems meeting metaneeds are corrected through the various modalities developed from the human potential movement.

STRESS AND COPING IN THE ELDERLY: A CLINICAL PARADIGM

A second way to organize the data gathered during the psychogeriatric evaluation is the psychodynamic paradigm, based on the pioneering work of Goldfarb[54,55] and expanded upon by me.[25,41,48,56–58] The elderly experience a variety of stresses

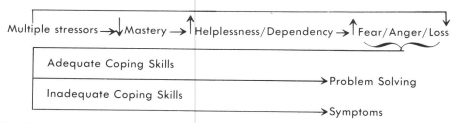

Fig. 4-1. Stress and coping in the elderly. With permission from Goldfarb AI: Clinical perspectives. In Simon A, Epstein LJ (eds): Aging in Modern Society: Psychiatric Research Report No. 23. Washington: American Psychiatric Association, 1968, pp 170–178.

triggering a characteristic sequence of coping events (Figure 4-1). Some of these stresses are rather sudden and unpredictable. These are stresses that may happen to individuals at any age but are more likely to occur in the elderly. They are also more likely to be clustered in the elderly. A common denominator of these stresses is that they all involve loss, including losses in the social support system—loss of friends, spouse, parents, children, neighbors, workmates. These losses may occur through death, illness, institutionalization, or relocation. Other losses occur in social role, including the shift from institutionalized roles at first to tenuous and informal roles, as described by Rosow,[80] and finally to a lapse into rolelessness.[56] In addition, the inability of men to perform traditional gender role behaviors is another significant loss that has important ramifications for rehabilitation; men faced with severe physical illness or functional disability are more likely to become severely depressed than women.[51,59,60] There are also other losses, including loss of health, mobility, income, adequate housing, and adequate opportunities for leisure-time activities.

Another set of stresses result from the daily victimization that the elderly face,[25,41,48,56] including economic, physical, attitudinal, and role victimization. Included here are ageism and stereotyping, as well as inadequate pensions and health insurance, high food prices, the effects of inflation, crimes against person and property, and inadequate medical evaluation and intervention. These stresses have been discussed in more depth elsewhere.[25,41,48,56,61,62]

When faced with these stresses, the elderly must cope with the feelings engendered. At first, the older person experiences a diminished sense of mastery over the environment. This decreasing mastery is associated with feelings of loss of control of one's destiny and over one's internal and/or external environment. These feelings then stimulate feelings of increased helplessness and ambivalent feelings about dependency. This sense of helplessness is often reinforced by health care workers because of stereotyping and ageism, the inappropriate adoption of the "sick" role[63,64] (which is antithetical to adequate intervention in a rehabilitation setting), and the power differential inherent in the interpersonal relationship between patient and therapist.[38,45,46] These feelings then stimulate the two underlying stress affects mediated by the general adaptation syndrome.[65] These affects (fight and flight) are experienced as feelings of anger or fear. The amount of anger and fear experienced by the older patient is largely determined by previous life experiences as well as the specific nature of the stress. In addition, anger and fear become separate affects as people age, so that the older patient experiences a third stress affect, loss.

The older person must then diminish the discomfort of these dysphoric feelings. The older person who has adequate coping skills will be able to regain a sense of mastery, avoid lapsing into a state of helplessness, ventilate feelings appropriately, and bring cognitive, problem-solving, and adaptive skills and psychogenic defense mechanisms into play. The dysphoric feelings are then minimized and the person alloplastically manipulates the environment.

However, if the person is unable to bring adequate coping skills into play, psychologic symptoms will develop. These symptoms (Figure 4-2) are largely dependent upon the underlying affective experience. For example, the behavioral manifestation of anger is rage and physical assault; the behavioral manifestation of fear is panic. Various mixtures of these two affects lead to other psychopathologic symptoms. The more loss the person experiences, the less manifest anxiety will be evident. In addition, if the person has always been narcissistic and oriented toward the body, somatization will be a concomitant symptom, regardless of the nature of the specific symptoms.

There are three groups of older people who have difficulty coping and are likely to develop psychologic symptoms. The major group includes those elderly who have previously been able to cope well with stress; however, because of the severity of this stress and/or the clustering of stress, their coping mechanisms have become overwhelmed, and their coping abilities have broken down. A second group of individuals also previously coped well with stress; however, because of brain failure they have become unable to bring previously acquired coping skills into play and thus develop symptoms. These symptoms are usually an exaggeration of either the underlying affects or the individual's premorbid personality and coping mechanisms. The third group is the smallest but causes the most difficulty, and its members are the most difficult to treat. These are older people who have never been able to cope with stress, including older people with a past history of personality disorders[25] or other major psychopathology.

This paradigm has many important implications for physical therapists. Most

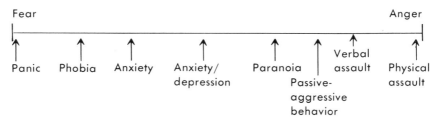

Fig. 4-2. Psychopathologic symptoms in the elderly and their place on the fear–anger continuum. With permission from Solomon K: The elderly patient. In Spittell JA Jr (ed): Clinical Medicine, Vol. 12. Psychiatry. Harper & Row, Hagerstown, Md., 1982, pp. 1–14.

obvious is that loss of function is a very great stress at any age. There is a real loss of mastery, not only because the individual is no longer able to manage activities of daily living, but also because the stressful events themselves are not under the control of the individual in any way. Dependency on others is a reality issue, as is true helplessness, thus leading to conflict between real dependency and clinical goals that emphasize autonomy, independence, and minimization of disability. The sense of vulnerability engenders feelings of fear of recurrence of the underlying trauma or illness. Some patients feel anger at themselves for slow progression in therapy or for getting sick, or anger at God or at health care personnel for not being able to reverse problems and return the patient to the premorbid state. Loss of functioning requires that the individual grieve as he or she would grieve over any other loss. In addition, the older person must cope with the continuous stresses of ageism manifested in the health care system that reinforce learned helplessness and depressive symptomatology.[38,45,46,56]

COMMON PSYCHOPATHOLOGIC SYNDROMES IN THE ELDERLY

Adjustment Disorders

Adjustment disorders are virtually ubiquitous in the elderly. Such disorders are a response to any stress, and they are especially common following a major physical illness that requires rehabilitation. An adjustment disorder is a time-limited and mildly exaggerated form of the individual's usual coping mechanisms as the person experiences a wide variety of mood changes, including euphoria and elation, sadness, anger, self-blame, irritability, anxiety, hostility, and a variety of somatic complaints. The person's mood remains quite labile, and shifts within this range of feelings occur with minimal external or internal provocation. However, as the person begins to cope with the stress, these symptoms begin to improve, usually within days or weeks, which differentiates this disorder from other pathologic symptoms that tend to remain stable or get worse. The adjustment disorder differs from normative coping in that the individual acknowledges difficulty coping or the process of coping seems to become stalled for several weeks. The treatment of the adjustment disorder is psychotherapeutic and sociotherapeutic.

Affective Disorders

Affective disorders (depression and mania) are the most common major psychopathologic syndromes in the elderly. Estimates of the after-age-65 incidence of depression usually are approximately 30 percent, and depression accounts for 68 percent of psychiatric hospitalizations in the elderly.[66] Approximately 14 percent of the elderly suffer from depression at some time.[67] Depression is manifested by sad mood (or its equivalent) and various vegetative disturbances. There is a change in appetite (usually loss but occasionally increase) and a change in the sleep cycle (usually difficulty falling asleep, difficulty remaining asleep, and early morning awakening, but occasionally hypersomnia). The person demonstrates either psychomotor agitation or retardation and may complain of anxiety, weakness, or feeling slowed up, but not of sadness. The patient feels fatigued, even after adequate sleep, and feels lacking in the energy or the motivation for rehabilitation and other tasks. The patient feels guilty and blames himself or herself for these problems. The patient has difficulty concentrating and demonstrates a cognitive disturbance manifested by a disturbance of recent memory and immediate recall, concrete thinking, pervasive doubt, and what I have described as "viewing the world through gray-colored glasses." In addition, the depressed individual manipulates self and others into situations that will guarantee failure[68, 69] and then internalizes the guilt and anger at others who do not respond to these failure-invoking manipulations.

The severely depressed person may verbalize suicidal feelings, ideation, or plans. As suicide is one of the leading causes of death in the elderly, the examiner must always ask the patient about suicidal ideation. Some severely depressed individuals will also demonstrate a variety of psychotic symptoms, including delusions and hallucinations.

It is important to differentiate depression from an adjustment disorder, a relatively easy task except early in the course of the disorder. People with adjustment disorders with sad mood will gradually improve over time; those with depression will get worse. In addition, the depression may mimic a dementia (pseudodementia)[70] and must be differentiated from other causes of brain failure. The treatment of depression is psychopharmacologic, psychotherapeutic, and sociotherapeutic.

Mania is much less common in the elderly than it is in younger patients and may have either an organic or psychologic foundation. In some ways it is the extreme opposite of depression, as the manic individual's mood is elated or euphoric. The patient demonstrates extreme impulsivity, diminished need for sleep, increased energy, psychomotor agitation, and rapid speech. Many manic individuals are quite hostile and may be overtly paranoid. Some also demonstrate hallucinations or delusions. The treatment of mania also is psychopharmacologic, psychotherapeutic, and sociotherapeutic.

Alcoholism and Chemical Dependence

Approximately 25 percent of people over the age of 65 are at risk for developing alcoholism or chemical dependency. A majority of these individuals are reactive alcoholics who also suffer from severe depression. The drinking or abuse of drugs almost always begins after a major stress with loss. The use of alcohol or other drugs is clearly for self-medication of dysphoric affects. The pattern of drinking, in particular, is frequently different from that of younger alcoholics, as older reactive alcoholic men tend to drink alone to ward off feelings of depression, loneliness, and dependency. Older reactive alcoholic women often drink in the company of others and use alcohol to allow them to express feelings of anger and hostility. The treatment of alcoholism and chemical dependency first involves treatment of the underlying depression, followed by appropriate psychotherapy, sociotherapy, and attendance at an Alcoholics Anonymous–type support organization.

Brain Failure

Approximately 6.2 percent of the elderly develop symptoms of brain failure.[71] As one fourth of these individuals have a reversible condition, it is necessary that health workers not label the older patient with cognitive impairment as having an irreversible dementia. Depressive pseudodementia is only one of the common causes of reversible brain failure (or pseudosenility);[70] others are drug toxicity, malnutrition, infection, cerebral edema, and cardiovascular disease. The major cause of irreversible dementia is Alzheimer's disease, but other major causes are multiinfarct dementia, alcoholic dementia, tertiary neurosyphilis, head trauma, and cerebrovascular accident. The symptoms of brain failure are either primary (based on the neurologic dysfunction itself) or secondary (symptoms that include the individual's attempt to cope with and adapt to the primary symptoms, using the coping mechanisms described above). Brain failure is discussed in more detail in Chapter 5.

Paraphrenia

Paraphrenia is a paranoid psychosis that develops for the first time in old age in the absence of an organic cause of brain failure. It affects approximately 1 to 2 percent of the elderly and is manifested by paranoid delusions usually limited to only small segments of the patient's life and allowing the patient to function in the usual way. Treatment is a combination of pharmacotherapy and psychosocial interventions.

Other Psychopathology

Personality disorders affect approximately 5 percent of the elderly[25] and are lifelong maladaptive interpersonal behavior patterns that may become evident for the first time or intensified in old age. Neuroses, phobias, and anxiety disorders are syndromes that are rare in the elderly. When they do occur, they are frequently indicative of an underlying depression or organic problem. The treatment of these disorders is psychotherapeutic. Sexual dysfunctions may also occur for the first time in old age; besides demythologization and education, treatment follows the techniques developed by Masters and Johnson.[72]

PRINCIPLES OF INTERVENTION

The goal of intervention is to change symptoms into adequate coping and adaptation by reversing the psychodynamic schema noted above. Most of this reversal can be accomplished by members of the rehabilitation team, utilizing generalist skills. As Rogers[73] has pointed out, the major hallmarks of a good psychophysical therapist are not technical skills but rather empathy (the ability to psychologically put oneself in the other person's place), unconditional positive regard (the ability to accept the patient as she or he is; this is not the same as liking the patient), and genuineness (accepting yourself as you are).

The first step in therapy is a direct attack on the symptoms. If the person has psychotic symptoms (mania, delusions, hallucinations), catastrophic reactions, or organically based agitation that is not controlled by nonpharmacologic measures, antipsychotic medication (Table 4-2) is indicated. Antipsychotic medications should not be used to treat symptoms of anxiety, as there is no evidence that these medications are efficacious for such problems.[74] Nor should they be used in the treatment of organically based symptoms until the underlying cause of the symptoms are elucidated. If the patient meets the criteria for a diagnosis of major depressive disorder, antidepressant medication (Table 4-3) is indicated. Antidepressants should not be used in the treatment of anxiety nor for adjustment disorders, sadness, or grief reactions. If the patient is manic, lithium is the treatment of choice.

If the older person demonstrates phobic, compulsive, or obsessive symptoms, the use of behavior modification techniques is indicated.[75,76] Sexual dysfunctions may be treated by sexual therapies developed by Masters and Johnson.[72] Hypnosis may also be used for specific neurotic symptoms. A variety of nonpharmacologic techniques may be used in the treatment of anxiety. For episodic anxiety, the breathing exercises developed for use in Lamaze childbirth[77] are of help. For more continuous anxiety or tension, relaxation exercises, such as used in behavior modification or Lamaze childbirth, may be of help. For some patients regular

Table 4-2. Antipsychotic Drugs

Phenothiazines
  Aliphatic
    Chlorpromazine (Thorazine)
    Promazine (Sparine)
    Triflupromazine (Vesprin)
  Piperidine
    Thioridazine (Mellaril)
    Mesoridazine (Serentil)
    Piperacetazine (Quide)
  Piperazine
    Prochlorperazine   (Compazine)
    Trifluoperazine (Stelazine)
    Butaperazine (Repoise)
    Perphenazine (Trilafon)
    Fluphenazine (Prolixin, Permitil)
    Acetophenazine (Tindal)
Thioxanthines
  Chlorprothixene (Taractan)
  Thiothixene (Navane)
Butyrophenones
  Haloperidol (Haldol)
Dihydroindolones
  Molindone (Moban, Lidone)
Dibenzoxazepines
  Loxapine (Loxitane, Daxolin)

Table 4-3. Antidepressant Drugs

Tricyclics
  Iminobenzyls
    Imipramine (Tofranil, Presamine, Imavate, Janimine, W.D.D., SK-Pra-
        mine)
    Trimipramine (Surmontyl)
    Desipramine (Norpramin, Pertofrane)
  Dibenzoheptadienes
    Amitriptyline (Elavil, Endep)
    Nortriptyline (Aventyl, Pamelor)
    Protriptyline (Vivactyl)
  Dibenzoxepins
    Doxepin (Sinequan, Adapin)
  Dibenzoxazepines
    Amoxapine (Asendin)
Tetracyclics
  Maprotiline (Ludiomil)
Monoamine oxidase inhibitors
  Isocarboxazid (Marplan)
  Tranylcypromine (Parnate)
  Phenelzine (Nardil)

strenuous physical exercise, transcendental meditation, yoga, massage, sex, or biofeedback may also be of benefit in mastering anxiety. Because of the unproven efficacy of benzodiazepines[74, 78] (Table 4-4) and other antianxiety agents such as hydroxyzine or meprobamate,[74, 79] these drugs probably have no place in the treatment of the elderly. However, the sedation caused by benzodiazepines may be helpful as an adjunct treatment for chronic anxiety if nonpharmacologic interventions have not been successful.

Following the direct attack on symptoms, the therapist next helps the patient ventilate the underlying affect. This involves giving the patient permission to feel fear, anger, or loss and to verbalize these feelings. Permission must be especially given to dependent individuals who are afraid of antagonizing the therapist if they get angry at the therapist. It should be made clear that it is "okay" to be angry at members of the rehabilitation team and to direct this anger at them rather than toward self. Patients who are particularly labile in expressing affect must learn how to channel affect into verbal communication. Those who do not express affect must be pushed to do so.

The next step in therapy is to diminish helplessness and dependency. In part, this process utilizes the techniques of rehabilitation. The patient must internalize feelings that counter helplessness and dependency. Aside from the work of the re-

Table 4-4. Benzodiazepines

Chlordiazepoxide (Librium, Libritabs, SK-Lygen)
Diazepam (Valium)
Oxazepam (Serax)
Clorazepate (Tranxene, Azene)
Prazepam (Vestran, Centrax)
Lorazepam (Ativan)
Halazepam (Paxipam)
Alprazolam (Xanax)

habilitation team, one way of accomplishing this is to give the patient graded behavioral tasks with guaranteed success to build up a hierarchy of behaviors.

Regaining mastery requires that the patient have control over his or her life. That requires choice and options. The patient must be made to understand that she or he is responsible for his or her own behavior; at first, this may be the patient's only expectation. The patient should be allowed to make all decisions for herself or himself, including decisions regarding clothing, menu, visitors, activities, and therapeutic goals. The patient should not be cut off from his or her network, but must use this network to help maintain autonomy and mastery. The older person must be encouraged to take risks and to try out new options, including options that may not be comfortable for the therapist yet are comfortable for the patient.

Whenever possible, the specific stresses must be reversed. It is important to realize that the specific physical stress may have ramifications involving the entire spectrum of stresses felt by the older person. For example, the stress of hemiparesis also involves the stresses of involuntary retirement, changed relationship with spouse and children, loss of ability to perform leisure activities, and financial problems.

For the older person who has previously functioned well, rehabilitation and psychosocial support are frequently all the therapy that is necessary. For the older person with a lifelong history of inadequate coping or who wishes to grow, long-term psychiatric intervention is indicated. If the problems are primarily intrapsychic, a form of individual psychotherapy is the treatment of choice. For those who are psychologically minded, an insight-oriented psychotherapy (psychoanalysis, psychoanalytically oriented psychotherapy, Gestalt therapy, transactional analysis, client-centered psychotherapy, or existential therapy) is the treatment of choice, augmented with a movement therapy, such as Feldenkrais or dance therapy, massage therapy, neurolinguistic programming, or art therapy. If the problems are primarily interpersonal, group psychotherapy or marital therapy is indicated. For those individuals unable to work within an insight-oriented mode, the same techniques modified for supportive psychotherapy are helpful. These various therapies require appropriate members of the treatment team to adopt specialist roles.

CONCLUSION

Adequate treatment of the elderly begins with adequate evaluation. Adequate evaluation and intervention have cognitive, skill, and affective components.[22–23] The cognitive component is the knowledge of what it is that one needs to do; the skill is having the tools; the affective components are the awareness of the therapist's attitude toward older people and working with them and how this relates to the stereotype of the elderly, all translated into daily interactions.

This chapter has examined these various issues and has offered therapists an outline of a comprehensive psychosocial assessment of the elderly, and a general guideline for assessment and intervention, in the hope that physical therapists will utilize these tools in their work with older people who require physical therapy.

REFERENCES

1. Solomon K: An objection to the use of the term "acting-out." Hosp Commun Psychiatry 27:733,1976.
2. MacKenzie TB, Rosenberg SD, Bergen BJ, et al: The manipulative patient: An interactional approach. Psychiatry 41:264–271, 1978.
3. Offer D, Sabshin M: Normality: Theoretical and Clinical Concepts of Mental Health. Basic Books, New York, 1966.
4. Goffman E: Encounters. Bobbs-Merrill, Indianapolis, Ind., 1961, p. 84.
5. Scheff TJ: Schizophrenia as ideology. Schizophr Bull No 2:15–19, 1970.
6. Goffman E: Asylums. Doubleday, New York, 1961.
7. Rosenhan DL: On being sane in insane places. Science 179:250–258, 1973.
8. Maslow AH: The Farther Reaches of Human Nature. Viking, New York, 1971.
9. American Psychiatric Association: Diagnostic and Statistical Manual of Mental Disorders, 3rd ed. Washington, American Psychiatric Association, 1980.
10. Graham DT: Health, disease, and the mind–body problem: Linguistic parallelism. Psychosom Med 29:52–71, 1967.
11. Cohen RE: The collaborative co-professional: Developing a new mental health role. Hosp Commun Psychiatr 24:242–246, 1973.
12. Harris M, Solomon K: Roles of the community mental health nurse. J Psychiatr Nurs Mental Health Services 15:35–39, 1977.
13. Howard M: The community mental health nurse and geropsychiatry. Presented at the 32nd Annual Meeting of the Gerontological Society, Washington, D.C., 26 Nov 1979.
14. Gottesman LE, Ishizaki B, MacBride SM: Service management—Plan and concept in Pennsylvania. Gerontologist 19:379–385, 1979.
15. Ishizaki B, Gottesman LE, MacBride SM: Determinants of model choice for service management systems. Gerontologist 19:385–388, 1979.
16. Pons SL: Roles of the community geropsychiatric social worker. Presented at the 32nd Annual Meeting of the Gerontological Society, Washington, D.C., 26 Nov 1979.
17. Romaniuk M: A look at the psychologist's role on a community geropsychiatry team. Presented at the 32nd Annual Meeting of the Gerontological Society, Washington, D.C., 26 Nov 1979.
18. Smith FS: Definition of a generalist. Albany, Capital District Psychiatric Center, Mimeo, 1972.
19. Solomon K: The geropsychiatrist and the delivery of mental health services in the community. Presented at the 32nd Annual Meeting of the Gerontological Society, Washington, D.C., 26 Nov 1979.
20. Solomon K: The roles of the psychiatric resident on a community psychiatry team. Psychiatr Q 54:67–76, 1982.
21. Rapoport M, Cahn B: The geriatric AHEC at the University of Maryland: A model for geriatric education. In: Geriatric Education, ed. Steel K. Collamore Press, Lexington, Mass., 1981, pp 201–207.
22. Grabowski BL, Kappelman MM, Cahn B, Solomon K: Geropsychiatric education in an interdisciplinary setting. Presented at the 33rd Annual Meeting of the Gerontological Society of America, San Diego, Calif., 22 Nov 1980.

23. Grabowski BL, Kappelman MM, Cahn B, Solomon K: Geropsychiatric education in an interdisciplinary setting. Gerontol Geriatr Educ 3:29–35, 1982.
24. Ayd FJ Jr: Treatment-resistant patients: A moral, legal and therapeutic challenge. In: Rational Psychopharmacotherapy and the Right of Treatment, ed. Ayd FJ Jr. Ayd Medical Communications, Baltimore, Md., 1975, pp 37–61.
25. Solomon K: Personality disorders in the elderly. In: Personality Disorders: Diagnosis and Management, 2nd ed., ed. Lion JR. Williams and Wilkins, Baltimore, Md., 1981, pp 310–338.
26. Cicero: On old age (44 B.C.), In: Selected Works, transl. Grant M. Penguin, Baltimore, Md., 1960, pp 213–247.
27. Weiss JAM: The natural history of antisocial attitudes. What happens to psychopaths? J Geriatr Psychiatry 6:236–242, 1973.
28. Adams FD: Physical Diagnosis. Williams and Wilkins, Baltimore, Md., 1958, pp 1–16.
29. Delp MH: Study of the patient. In: Major's Physical Diagnosis, ed. Delp MH, Manning RT. Saunders, Philadelphia, Pa., 1968, pp 13–26.
30. Friedland E: Clinical Clerk Case Study Outline. State University of New York at Buffalo, 1967.
31. Judge RD, Zuidema GD: Physical Diagnosis. A Physiologic Approach. Little, Brown, Boston, Mass., 1963, pp 9–25.
32. Menninger KA: A Manual for Psychiatric Case Study, 2nd ed. Grune and Stratton, New York, 1962.
33. Stevenson I, Sheppe WM Jr: The psychiatric examination. In: American Handbook of Psychiatry, Vol. I, 2nd ed., ed. Arieti S. Basic Books, New York, 1974, pp 1157–1180.
34. MacKinnon RA: Psychiatric history and mental status examination. In: Comprehensive Textbook of Psychiatry, Vol. I, 3rd ed., ed. Kaplan HI, Freedman AM, Sadock BJ. Williams and Wilkins, Baltimore, Md., 1980, pp 906–920.
35. Kendell RE, Brockington IF, Leff JP: Prognostic implications of six alternative definitions of schizophrenia. Arch Gen Psychiatry 36:25–31, 1979.
36. Folstein MD, Folstein SE, McHugh PR: Mini-Mental State: A practical method for grading the cognitive state of patients for the clinician, J Psychiatr Res 12:189–198, 1975.
37. McTavish DG: Perceptions of old people. A review of research methodologies and findings. Gerontologist 11 (Part II):90–101, 1971.
38. Solomon K: Social antecedents of learned helplessness in the health care setting. Gerontologist 22:282–287, 1982.
39. Solomon K, Vickers R: Stereotyping the elderly: Changing the attitudes of clinicians. Presented at the 33rd Annual Meeting of the Gerontological Society of America, San Diego, Calif., 25 Nov 1980.
40. Solomon K, Vickers R: Stereotyping the elderly: Further research on changing the attitudes of clinicians. Presented at the 34th Annual Meeting of the Gerontological Society of America and 10th Annual Meeting of the Canadian Association on Gerontology, Toronto, 10 Nov 1981.
41. Solomon K: Victimization by health professionals and the psychologic response of the elderly. In: The Abuse and Maltreatment of the Elderly, ed. Kosberg JI. Wright-PSG, Littleton, Mass., in press.
42. Solomon K, Vickers R: Attitudes of health workers toward old people. J Am Geriatr Soc 27:186–191, 1979.
43. Butler RN: Why Survive: Being Old in America. Harper and Row, New York, 1975, pp 174–259.
44. O'Dowd M, Zofnass J: Behavioral implications of attitudes toward the elderly. Pre-

sented at a regional meeting of the World Psychiatric Association, New York, 31 Oct 1981.

45. Solomon K: Social antecedents of learned helplessness in the health care setting. Presented at the 31st Annual Meeting of the Gerontological Society, Dallas, Tex., 19 Nov 1978.

46. Solomon K: Social antecedents of learned helplessness of the elderly in the health care setting. In: Sociological Research Symposium Proceedings (IX), ed. Lewis EP, Nelson LD, Scully DH, et al. Virginia Commonwealth University, Richmond, Va., 1979, pp 188–192.

47. Tuckman J, Lorge I: Attitudes toward old people. J Soc Psychol 37:249–260, 1953.

48. Solomon K: The elderly patient. In: Clinical Medicine, Vol. 12. Psychiatry, ed. Spittell JA Jr. Harper & Row, Hagerstown, Md., 1982, pp 1–14.

49. Shagass C: The medical model in psychiatry. In: Hormones, Behavior, and Psychopathology, ed. Sachar EJ. Raven Press, New York, 1976, pp 291–300.

50. Exton-Smith AN, Overstall PW: Geriatrics. University Park Press, Baltimore, Md., 1979, pp 17–34.

51. Solomon K: The older man. In: Men in Transition: Theory and Therapy, ed. Solomon K, Levy NB. Plenum, New York, 1982, pp 205–240.

52. Vickers R: Needs assessment of the elderly and community geropsychiatry. Presented at the 32nd Annual Meeting of the Gerontological Society, Washington, D.C., 26 Nov 1979.

53. Mijuskovic B: Loneliness: An interdisciplinary approach. Psychiatry 40:113–132, 1977.

54. Goldfarb AI: Clinical perspectives. In: Aging in Modern Society. Psychiatric Research Report No. 23, ed. Simon A, Epstein LJ. American Psychiatric Association, Washington, D.C., 1968, pp 170–178.

55. Goldfarb AI: Minor maladjustments of the aged. In: American Handbook of Psychiatry, Vol. 3, 2nd ed., ed. Arieti S, Brody EB. Basic Books, New York, 1974, pp 820–860.

56. Solomon K: The depressed patient: Social antecedents of psychopathology in the elderly. J Am Geriatr Soc 29:14–18, 1981.

57. Solomon K, Zinke MR: Group psychotherapy with the depressed elderly. Presented at the 58th Annual Meeting of the American Orthopsychiatric Association, New York, 31 Mar 1981.

58. Solomon K: Alzheimer's Disease: The subjective experience of the patient. Presented at a regional meeting of the World Psychiatric Association, New York, 31 Oct 1981.

59. Solomon K: Psychosocial crises of older men. Presented at the 133rd Annual Meeting of the American Psychiatric Association, San Francisco, Calif., 7 May 1980.

60. Solomon K: The masculine gender role and its implications for the life expectancy of older men. J Am Geriatr Soc 29:297–301, 1981.

61. Block M, Sinnott, JD: The Battered Elder Syndrome: An Exploratory Study. University of Maryland, College Park, 1979.

62. Kosberg JI: The Abuse and Maltreatment of the Elderly. Wright-PSG, Littleton, Mass., in press.

63. Parsons T: The Social System. Free Press, New York, 1951, pp 428–473.

64. Wilson RN: The Sociology of Health: An Introduction. Random House, New York, 1970, pp 13–32.

65. Selye H: The Physiology and Pathology of Exposure to Stress. Acta, Montreal, 1950.

66. Ban TA: The treatment of depressed geriatric patients. Am J Psychother 32:93–104, 1978.

67. Blazer D, Williams CD: Epidemiology of dysphoria and depression in an elderly population. Am J Psychiatry 137:439–444, 1980.

68. Kovacs M, Beck AT: Maladaptive cognitive structures in depression. Am J Psychiatry 135:525–533, 1978.
69. Bonime W: The psychodynamics of neurotic depression. In: American Handbook of Psychiatry, Vol. 3, 1st. ed., ed. Arieti S. Basic Books, New York, 1966, pp 239–255.
70. Libow LS: Pseudo-senility: Acute and reversible organic brain syndromes. J Am Geriatr Soc 21:112–120, 1973.
71. Kay DWK: The epidemiology and identification of brain deficit in the elderly. In: Cognitive and Emotional Disturbance in the Elderly, ed. Eisdorfer C, Freidel RO. Year Book Medical Publishers, Chicago, Ill., 1977, pp 11–26.
72. Masters WH, Johnson VE: Human Sexual Inadequacy. Little, Brown, Boston, Mass., 1970.
73. Rogers CR: A theory of therapy, personality and interpersonal relationships as developed in client-centered framework. In: Psychology: A Study of a Science, ed. Koch S. McGraw-Hill, New York, 1959, pp 192–256.
74. Solomon K: Benzodiazepines and neurotic anxiety. Critique. NY State J Med 76:2156–2164, 1976.
75. Wolpe J: The Practice of Behavior Therapy. Pergamon Press, New York, 1969.
76. Shaefer HH, Martin PL: Behavioral Therapy. McGraw-Hill, New York, 1969.
77. Bing E: Six Practical Lessons for an Easier Childbirth. Bantam, New York, 1969, pp 36–52.
78. Solomon K, Hart R: Pitfalls and prospects in clinical research on antianxiety drugs: Benzodiazepines and placebo. A research review. J Clin Psychiatry 39:823–831, 1978.
79. Greenblatt DJ, Shader RI: Meprobamate: A study of irrational drug use. Am J Psychiatry 127:1297–1303, 1971.
80. Rosow I: Status and role change through the life span. In: Handbook of Aging and the Social Sciences, ed. Birstock RH, Sharas E. Van Nostrand Reinhold, New York, 1976, pp. 457–482.

5 | Alzheimer's Disease and the Confused Patient

Nancy L. Mace
Sue R. Hardy
Peter V. Rabins

The rehabilitation therapist (physical or occupational therapist) is often called on to care for elderly patients with symptoms of impaired thinking or personality change associated with cognitive decline. We believe that the rehabilitation therapist's role in the care of such patients is important both in assessment of patient function and in assisting the patient to remain as independent as possible. This chapter briefly describes dementing illnesses and their diagnosis. We also discuss specific issues that commonly arise in the care of patients with dementing illnesses.

Although it has long been recognized that some individuals develop significant intellectual decline in later life, there has been disagreement over the nature and the inevitability of this decline. In the past few years, however, significant advances have been made in distinguishing normal intellectual age changes from diseases causing cognitive decline and in understanding the prevalence and etiology of the dementing illnesses.

Approximately 80 percent of those who live into very late life remain cognitively intact. However, in 1980 an estimated 2 million Americans had developed a senile dementia.[1] Approximately one third (usually those most seriously ill and without family support) were institutionalized. Another 11 percent may reside in boarding homes and similar settings. More than half the impaired individuals were cared for at home, usually by a spouse or adult child.[2] In 1981 the cost of nursing home care for patients with these illnesses exceeded 10.5 billion dollars.[3] Such figures indicate the impact of the dementing disorders.

Significant disagreement still exists about specific cognitive changes in normal aging. However, it is generally agreed that slower response time and slight memory deterioration (what has been termed "benign senescent forgetfulness") occur.[4] These changes interfere minimally with function. Such normal changes may be difficult to distinguish from the earliest symptoms of a disease process, but the differences become clinically obvious as the patient's level of function significantly declines.

DEMENTIA

A variety of terms have been used to describe the intellectual decline in late life. They include "acute" or "chronic" organic brain syndrome, "senility," and Alzheimer's disease. Confusion over definitions of terms has led to misinformation about prognosis and treatment, and it is therefore important to review the generally accepted terminology.

Dementia is a *global decline in intellectual function from a previous level occurring in clear consciousness.* This decline from previous levels must affect *several areas* of mental function, for example, memory, language, praxis (motor abilities), and judgment. These patients are awake, alert, and aware of their surroundings.[5]

Delirium is defined as *a decline in level of intellectual function in clouded consciousness.* Although they may be either drowsy or agitated, delirious patients are not alert or fully aware of their surroundings and have difficulty shifting and maintaining a focus of attention. Clinically, delirium is often seen as having a more abrupt or more recent onset than dementia, and function often fluctuates over hours or days; thus the term "acute organic brain syndrome" was used to refer to delirium.

Both delirium and dementia are syndromes, sets of symptoms that may be caused by a variety of diseases.

Alzheimer's disease accounts for about 50 percent of the cases of dementia. Another 20 percent of cases are diagnosed as multiinfarct dementia, and 20 percent of patients are believed to have both diseases.[6] The remaining 10 percent of cases are caused by a variety of rare conditions, including metabolic disorders (e.g., thyroid dysfunction), structural problems of the brain (e.g., normal pressure hydrocephalus, brain tumors, subdural hematoma), infectious disease (e.g., tuberculosis, tertiary suphilis), toxins (e.g., metal poisoning or alcoholism), degenerative diseases (e.g., Huntington's disease, Parkinson's disease, Pick's disease), autoimmune diseases, and psychiatric disorders (notably depression). About 10 percent of the patients seen[7] have reversible or treatable dementing illnesses.

Although the majority of the patients have a nonreversible dementia, many can be helped. The rehabilitation therapist can play a significant role in the care of such persons and their families by devising practical interventions that improve the quality of life for the patient and family or caregiver.

Alzheimer's disease is an irreversible, slowly progressive illness ending in death 4 to 15 (average 7) years after onset. The illness may be described as having three stages,[8] although the course is gradual, and many patients follow different courses. Symptoms of memory loss and sometimes personality change predominate in the first stage. These patients are usually still able to provide their own personal care, to socialize, and to function normally in many areas. They may be aware of their plight, and supportive psychotherapy may help them to adjust to the illness.

In the second stage memory loss worsens and aphasia, apraxias, and agnosia are increasingly evident. Aphasia is a disorder of language that often first appears as a difficulty in naming objects (anomia) but later is characterized by a misuse of words (e.g., "spool" for "spoon" or "fork" for "pen"). Apraxia, the inability to perform a learned motor movement although strength is intact, may first show up as difficulty in writing, in dressing, or in complex actions such as setting a table or knitting. Agnosia is the inability to know or recognize. There are many specific agnosias—for example, of faces or places, the inability to recognize objects, or seeing two objects at once. The patient in this second stage may have a lower tolerance for stress, may change eating patterns, may have difficulty walking, and may suffer disruption of sleep–wake cycles.

In the third and final stage, the patient becomes incontinent, bedfast, and severely aphasic. Strange sounds or single words may be produced. Alzheimer's disease patients have a shortened life expectancy. Death is often from a secondary condition such as pneumonia or a urinary tract infection, although this does not explain all early deaths.

The diagnosis of Alzeheimer's disease is based on the history of a gradually progressive dementia and on the elimination of other possible causes. Evidence from a CAT scan, while supportive, is not definitive. Based on autopsy studies of clinical course, it is now believed that Alzheimer's disease of both early-onset (presenile) and late-onset (senile dementia) type are the same or very similar diseases.

Multiinfarct dementia is the cumulative result of a number of cerebral infarcts that may be individually too small to be clinically observed. Multiinfarct dementia usually presents a history of a stepwise progression (abrupt, intermittent worsening of symptoms), in contrast to the gradual progression of Alzheimer's disease. A history of diabetes, hypertension, and heart disease is often present. Multiinfarct dementia is a potentially preventable or treatable disease. However, in clinical practice a number of patients are seen who continue to deteriorate. Research into the treatment and prevention of stroke should reduce the number of such patients. (Cerebral arteriosclerosis was for some time considered to cause dementia by reducing the oxygen supply to the brain, and a variety of treatments designed to increase blood flow or improve blood oxygenation were proposed. It is now clear that reduced blood and oxygen supplies to the brain rarely cause dementia, and treatments designed to improve blood flow or blood oxygenation have not been found to be helpful.)

Depression is a cause of dementia in a significant number of elderly people and should never be overlooked as the primary cause of dementia. Although an "understandable" depression at the onset of the dementing illness is seen in some patients, in others the depression is primary. A depressive illness usually includes vegetative symptoms of weight loss, disturbance of sleep patterns, and depressive delusions. When the depressive illness is treated, the dementia will resolve or improve.[9]

A dementia often develops in patients with Parkinson's disease, particularly in the late stages of the disease.

Korsakoff's syndrome is seen most commonly in patients with a history of alcoholism. It is characterized by an inability to form new memories, although other intellectual functions remain intact.

Patients with an existing dementing illness are especially vulnerable to developing a delirium, and this should be considered whenever an impaired patient worsens suddenly. The delirious patient may misinterpret reality, have false ideas or hallucinations, have incoherent speech, either sleepiness in the daytime or wakefulness at night, and either increased or decreased physical or motor activity. Delirium may be caused by a range of illnesses, such as pneumonia, urinary tract infection, congestive heart failure, malnutrition, dehydration, or even constipation. Medication is also a common cause of delirium (see Chapter 6). Thus when a patient displays intermittent intellectual impairment or memory disturbance of sudden onset, a delirium should be suspected and the underlying cause identified and treated.

In the past, funding policies, the individual attitudes of some professionals, and the chronic course of the dementing illnesses led to a reluctance to commit resources to individuals with dementia. Because resources are finite and value judgments must be made regarding their distribution, the individual therapist who is interested in the care of these patients may be discouraged from helping such persons. There are other problems the therapist may encounter as well. The rehabilitation specialist in an acute care facility may be pressured to help patients in a limited period of time. Therapists may be faced with unrealistic requests for a cure from the medical team or the family. In spite of such factors, the continuing care of these patients is a rewarding field for the therapist and can improve the quality of daily life for the patient.

THE FAMILY

The myth that the American family abandons its old and ill has been clearly disproven by Shanas.[10] Families do care for their elderly, often at great cost to themselves. The therapist may find the strength and resilience of family members to be one of the most rewarding aspects of caring for these patients (see Chapter 7).

DIAGNOSIS

The first step in intervention with the patient with an impairment in thinking is a thorough evaluation to determine its type (dementia or delirium).[11] A search for its cause should be undertaken and other medical conditions treated (as much as possible). A complete assessment should yield the following information:

1. Nature and cause of the illness or illnesses and their potential for treatment;
2. Nature and extent of the disability and the areas of spared function;
3. Social and psychologic resources and limitations;
4. Prognosis.

A patient with confusion and declining intellectual function should be given a complete physical and neurologic examination. A detailed history should be taken and a mental status examination done. We have found the Mini-Mental State Examination[12] (MMSE) to be a reliable instrument that reveals memory impairment, aphasia, and apraxia (see also Chapter 4).

Persons suffering from difficulty in thinking are often able to function more independently when specific areas of spared function are identified and their environment modified to make best use of these areas. An Activities of Daily Living (ADL) evaluation will identify specific areas in which the patient needs assistance in order to make the most use of remaining abilities.

It has been our experience that family members and caregiving staff benefit from a careful explanation of the findings of the evaluation. For example, such findings show family members that the patient forgets an item as soon as a second item to be remembered is presented, or that a patient's slow gait is an apraxia rather than "laziness." The physical and/or the occupational therapist should participate in family conferences, since the therapist has observed the patient attempting such activities during the ADL assessment and since the therapist possesses the expertise needed to devise ways to maximize patient function.

ASSESSMENT AND INTERVENTION

Deficits may be more widespread with dementia than in other illnesses, such as brain trauma or stroke, but it may be difficult to differentiate among such illnesses. For example, a patient being treated for an apraxia may not be able to *remember* instructions or may not *understand* instructions, thereby failing a task that he or she is in fact able to do if the difficulties in comprehension are eliminated. However, an understanding of the nature of the impairment is essential for effective intervention.

An assessment must be based on a knowledge of the patient's environment. The therapist will find that *change is most successfully effected in the environment rather than in the patient;* it is helpful to keep this focus in mind as interventions are devised.

The ADL evaluation should describe the extent of self-care in terms of cognitive ability as well as physical impairment. For example, in bathing, is the patient cognitively able to learn to use a grab bar? In toileting, is a raised toilet seat confusing? Can the patient use a familiar toilet but not a public rest room? An ADL evaluation may indicate that the patient can feed herself or himself when the plate is anchored or when weighted utensils give improved sensory clues. (Plastic, paper, or translucent utensils can increase confusion.)

The ADL evaluation can help the caregiver recognize that the patient can dress himself or herself but not select clothes, or operate zippers but not buttons. It will examine homemaking skills and identify impairments of judgment or sensation (for example, ability to mix hot and cold water). It will determine whether or not the patient is able to use a telephone, make change, or tell time.

Tests of memory, praxis, and language help to define limitations and resources (Does the patient understand instructions? Can she or he remember enough to follow a three-stage command?). The ADL evaluation will clarify the patient's ability to read and comprehend. Some patients can read aloud but are unable to act on the information they read.

It may fall to the therapist to determine if prescribed interventions for a physical disability may cause more problems for the patient who cannot remember or learn, or if alternative interventions can be divised. For example, a confused patient may perceive splints as a restraint and become upset or tear them off.

An important function of the ADL evaluation is the identification of hazards to the patient (discussed at length elsewhere[3]). When skills have been lost, the environment can often be adjusted to compensate for the loss: the temperature of a water heater can be adjusted, throw rugs removed, and stairs blocked off. Families often need specific instructions, such as: the patient cannot be left unsupervised, must be prevented from driving, or must wear an ID bracelet.

SENSORY DEFICITS

Sensory deficits must not be overlooked as a cause of dysfunction in a person who presents with confusion. Sensory deficits are common in the elderly, and sensory deprivation may present as depression or disorientation. The person with a dementia is unable to compensate for sensory decline and may misinterpret sensory information. This person may also be unable to learn to adjust to compensatory devices such as hearing aids, which amplify irrelevant sounds, or contact lenses following cataract surgery.

The assessment must differentiate between sensory loss and loss of comprehension (does the patient not hear you or not understand you?), agnosia (can the patient not see you or not assess what is seen?), loss of sensation, and loss of judgment.

One should ask the patient's family or nurse whether the patient has glasses or a hearing aid. They are often aware of sensory deficits that may otherwise be overlooked. Sensory impairments may become evident during an ADL evaluation or therapeutic intervention. One can ask patients directly if they can hear or if they can see specific objects. Tests should be requested if sensory loss is suspected. The rehabilitation therapist can assist in devising ways to help a demented person adjust to glasses or hearing aids. Sometimes the problem is as simple as informing the family that they (not the patient) must be responsible for checking the batteries in a hearing aid or keeping eyeglasses clean. In other cases large print, less background noise, and bright colors may be environmental modifications that help the patient to function more effectively.

MEMORY AND LEARNING

Memory impairment and the inability to learn new material are predominant features of dementia. Rehabilitation interventions can be more effective when the specific characteristics of the individual's forgetfulness are clearly defined. Some patients can retain certain types of information or can respond to memory cues in the environment. Many patients can respond to a one-stage command or single units of information but cannot handle more complex communications. This situation is easily evaluated and should be explained to everyone who will work with the patient. A patient who appears unable to follow instructions or complete a multistep task may in fact be able to do so if tasks are broken down into individual steps. For example, to help a patient transfer from wheelchair to toilet, give one-step instructions: "Put your hands on the rail." "Lean forward." "Push with your feet." Instructions should always be repeated exactly.

Patients may be better able to function if clues are given in several sensory modalities (for example, putting a toothbrush in a patient's hand and touching the limb that should be moved as the patient is instructed to brush his teeth).

Often a patient can perform a task at one time but not at another. Function frequently worsens in the evening. Therefore tests of function should be done at different times of day, and difficult or newly learned tasks scheduled for the patient's best times. The family or nursing staff may be able to chart the patient's daily variations. *Testing in an unfamiliar setting may give inaccurately negative results.* Confused patients often have difficulty orienting themselves in unfamiliar settings, which may distract them and cause them to function more poorly. Tests of function and efforts to teach new skills should be carried out, if possible, in the setting in which the patient will need to function, since information learned in one setting, such as a hospital, may not carry over to another setting, such as the home.

Patients (especially those seen in an acute-care hospital) may have a delirium superimposed on the dementia that additionally limits learning ability. This should be watched for and evaluated, since the patient may be more functional when the delirium clears.

Some patients are able to learn certain kinds of new information, such as the location of the bathroom in a new residence or the use of a prosthetic device, grab bar, cane, or walker; others will not be able to learn at all, and repeated efforts to teach them will frustrate both staff and patient. We have found that a 2-week trial is usually sufficient to determine whether or not a patient has the potential to learn new material.

Some patients can learn partially; for example, with consistent gentle reminders, they will use a grab bar. Many patients who never learn their way around a new environment do learn that a certain place is where they belong, so that wandering and complaints decrease. Studies of reality orientation[2] indicate that while it may be beneficial to frequently repeat to the patient information that is needed, little learning occurs or is retained. We tell the patients who we are, where they are, and what we are doing to them, and we repeat this information frequently, reassuring the patients that the therapist knows what is happening and will take care of them.

Everyone involved with a patient who has limited ability to learn must support the learning of new behaviors. Therefore staff and family involvement is essential. If family and nursing staff are not able to continue the teaching process at home, newly learned tasks are likely to be forgotten.

Everyone should use the same simplified one-step instructional phrases and give the same praise and encouragement. Families need to be told this explicitly.

Intermittent learning often confuses demented patients. For example, a patient learning to use a walker must be required to use it all the time. Positive reinforcement, the elimination of negative reinforcement, and the elimination of as much criticism as possible is important in working with a brain-injured person. It is not helpful to tell such patients that they are doing a task wrong because they lack the intellectual ability to remember how to do it correctly. The basic teaching approach would be to tell the patient what is being done right; suggest that the task be tried again; repeat instructions; give the patient the opportunity to rest between attempts; demonstrate the task; move the appropriate limbs; and give as many sensory clues as possible.

APRAXIA

Apraxias of dementia, particularly in Alzheimer's disease, are frequently more generalized than the apraxias seen in other conditions, such as a single stroke. Memory disorder or aphasia may interfere with the evaluation of specific apraxias. For example, patients may be able to feed themselves but be unable to understand or remember verbal instructions and therefore be unable to perform the same task in the evaluation setting. Direct observation in a familiar setting should replace verbal instruction.

Asking the patient to copy a simple diagram is a reliable test for even subtle apraxias and is helpful in separating symptoms of apraxia from other symptoms.

Apraxias often present as the inability to do a complex task. Breaking down such tasks into individual steps can help a patient remain independent. For example, step-by-step instructions will help a patient bathe. Often one part of a task, such as undoing a zipper, proves to be the stumbling block to independence in an area such as self-toileting. Explaining to family members that they must assist at this one point can prevent accidents and reduce the patient's frustration (an alternative is to try Velcro in place of the zipper). In some cases a task can be simplified. For example, patients who have difficulty using eating utensils may be able to use one eating utensil but become confused by the presence of several.

When an apraxia interferes with a specific function, patients may be unable to learn new skills to compensate. For example, patients may be unable to learn to use a walker. They may carry the walker, creating a hazard to themselves and others. It may be necessary to accept only limited improvement in such situations. The object should be to improve the quality of life for the patients. They may be safer and more mobile in a wheelchair than with a walker they cannot learn to use.

Often ingenious ways can be devised to use old skills to partially improve a patient's mobility or independence. A knowledge of the patient's past can help. Use familiar activities to initiate movements—for example, instruct a patient to "rock it like a baby," or "shake hands."

Apraxias can cause difficulty in swallowing. An ear, nose, and throat consultation should be obtained if choking, drooling of food, or dribbling occurs.

APHASIA

As with apraxia, other cognitive problems can complicate the assessment of aphasia. Some patients successfully conceal language problems so that an untrained observer or family member may not realize that the patient is aphasic. Failure to follow instructions can sometimes be misinterpreted as stubbornness. Confabulation, perseveration (repetition of a sound, word, or phrase) and other abnormalities of language are sometimes blamed on "old age," "living in the past," or an unpleasant personality. Thus aphasia should be specifically tested for. Most aphasic patients cannot repeat a phrase (for example, "This is a nice day in October") and often misname familiar objects. (Point to a watch, pen, or ring and ask the patient, "What do you call this?")

Communication is often possible even with severely aphasic patients.[13] Most patients communicate more successfully when they are relaxed; thus it is necessary to create a familiar, nonstressful atmosphere.

Words can be "filled in." We encourage family members to do so, since this seems to be less upsetting than forcing a patient to struggle to communicate. However, it is important to confirm that you are correctly understanding the patient. It is often possible to understand the meaning from the emotional content rather than the literal content. "I want to go home" may mean "I don't know where I am." Again, it is important to confirm with the patient the accuracy of your interpretation.

Watch the patient's nonverbal communications. If the patient is not listening to or understanding you, this may be clear from actions or facial expression. When working with a patient, watch his or her face: the patient may not be able to verbalize feelings of pain or fright.

When talking to a patient with a receptive aphasia or a dementia, first ascertain that you have the patient's attention and that she or he can hear you. Watch to see if the patient is paying attention to you. The patient who is distracted by activities in the room or who is upset may have difficulty focusing on what is being said.

Simplify information given to the confused person, and supplement verbal information with other environmental cues: give simple, one-stage instructions; repeat them; *wait* for the patient to respond. Confused people often take longer to respond, and it is important that neither therapist nor patient feel rushed. Confirm that the patient comprehends your instructions before continuing. Patients may reply "yes" when in fact they do not understand. Ask questions in a way that requires an answer that demonstrates comprehension. (Say, e.g., "Point to where it hurts.")

Demonstrate a physical activity or assist the patient in moving through an exercise. Give information in ways familiar to the patient. For example, instead of teaching exercises as such, ask the patient to do a familiar task that will exercise the target muscle group. Instead of saying, "Extend your arms," you may be more successful saying, "Reach for my hand."

AGNOSIA

Agnosia is frustrating both to professional staff and to family members. Patients may be unable to recognize family members or friends or to recognize their own room or own home. Agnosias can be confused with sensory disorders, memory loss, or aphasia. Often other sensory clues will help to orient the patient. For example, the patient who does not recognize a face may be able to recognize the person's voice. Familiar odors or possessions may help patients orient themselves. Environmental cues, such as the smell of food cooking, familiar furniture, or the texture of one's own blanket, should be gently called to the patient's attention.

CATASTROPHIC REACTIONS

Individuals with cognitive impairment may become emotionally distraught in the face of relatively minor stresses. Goldstein[14] has termed this behavior a "catastrophic reaction," and it is one of the most common problems that families report to us.[15] The patient may refuse to cooperate, argue, cry, resist assistance, or ignore the therapist. Some patients, when severely upset, may yell, scream, throw things, or strike those who attempt to intervene. In some cases such reactions are almost continuous.

A key principle in working with a confused patient is to avoid catastrophic reactions or to defuse them as early as possible when they occur. Teaching the family or staff how to recognize them early and how to react is important. Our clinical experience has shown that an understanding of catastrophic reactions is often the most important single factor in helping an impaired person remain at home. Those involved in caring for and relating to the patient must understand that much of the unpleasant behavior is a factor of brain injury and not willful behavior. Understanding is the first step in learning to respond to the patient's behavior constructively rather than in anger.

Catastrophic reactions are precipitated by

1. Misinterpretation of a request;
2. Misinterpretation of sensory information;
3. Cognitive overload (receiving too many sensory inputs simultaneously);

4. The inability to perform a task; and
5. Fatigue.

Restructuring of the patient's environment to avoid or limit these factors is an important part of maximizing patient function.

Give patients clear, simple information, one step at a time. Tell them where they are and what is being done for them. For example, say, "I am going to lift your arm for you," or "I am helping you unbutton your blouse." Avoid complex explanations, such as, "You have to go downstairs to the therapy room to practice with your walker so you will get better and go home." Reassure the patient that she or he is all right. Whenever possible, give information both verbally and visually. You may have to repeat the same information frequently.

Stand where a patient can see you. Avoid approaching and touching a patient from behind or allowing others to remain out of sight. Provide adequate lighting. If patients have sensory losses, remind them gently that they might have misinterpreted what they thought they saw or heard. Avoid arguing with the patients; instead, respond with empathy to their distress.

Reduce the amount of noise and activity going on around a confused, disoriented person. Whenever possible allow the patient to be in a familiar place when doing a difficult task. Reduce the number of places where the patient has to look for things, and reduce the number of choices the patient must make. (For example, limit the number of items of food on a plate.)

Recognize that what may once have been a simple task may now be impossible (such as tying shoes). Gently helping patients may be better than coaxing them to do such a task themselves. In a chronic condition, efforts to teach or encourage the patient will not bring back lost abilities; they will only humiliate the patient.

Schedule stressful tasks, such as learning of new skills, bathing, visiting, or other activities that you have observed to upset the patient, at times of day when a patient is at his or her best and is least fatigued.

Occasionally medications are used to help control catastrophic reactions, but only as a supplement to environmental modifications. Medication should not be used as a substitute for efforts to make the environment comprehensible to a confused person.

Catastrophic reactions are sometimes misinterpreted as characteristics of personality, particularly when a patient's premorbid personality included elements resembling the catastrophic behavior and when a patient's social functioning remains superficially intact. An important part of the training of staff and family members is to overcome this tendency to interpret catastrophic behavior as a controllable aspect of personality.

SUSPICIOUSNESS

Several factors contribute to the common phenomenon of excessive suspiciousness or suspicious uncooperativeness. Confused patients may easily misinterpret information or misinterpret procedures. For example, moving a patient's limbs for her or him may be misinterpreted as an attack or as sexual behavior. Forgetful patients mislay possessions, forget where items are, and misinterpret their absence as theft. The inability to make sense out of the environment and to remember can exacerbate and heighten normal behaviors of cautiousness.

However, some suspiciousness goes beyond misinterpretation and involves fixed delusions. When this situation occurs, it should be regarded as a factor of the brain disorder; it is usually not responsive to reason. Arguing with the patients or denying their feelings may precipitate a catastrophic reaction. Medication, judiciously used, may help with delusional ideas. Often it is equally important to reassure staff and family that the patient "cannot help" his or her behavior.

The therapist must take the time to establish rapport with the patient. This can be difficult for the therapist working in an acute-care hospital, where time with the patient is limited. However, gaining of the patient's trust is necessary to the success of interventions. Often a suspicious patient will cooperate with a person she or he trusts even when clearly confused or disoriented. One can empathize with the distress of persons who do not understand where they are or what is being done to them and who cannot remember what they are told. Respect for patients communicates itself no matter how ill the patients are. Taking time to listen to patients even when their speech is rambling and confused, visiting with patients about times past, and confirming that patients understand what the therapist is saying indicates that the therapist understands patient fears and anxieties and helps to establish trust.

APATHY

There are many reasons why a patient is apathetic or refuses to cooperate in treatment. The brain damage itself may cause apathy. Failure to understand instructions or frequent catastrophic reactions are often contributing factors. Older people are often afraid of falling, particularly when they are unsteady or have already experienced a fall.

Depression and delirium are frequently overlooked as causes of apathetic or even resistant behavior. Depression and delirium should be treated when identified. Confused, apathetic patients may have catastrophic reactions if they are addressed briskly or given firm orders. A good rapport, patience, and elimination of causes of catastrophic reactions is more effective.

SUMMARY

The rehabilitation team and physical therapy can play a valuable role in the care of chronically ill demented patients. As with any other condition, the first step in such care is an accurate diagnosis and ongoing medical supervision of the illness and other health problems. When this has been accomplished, the rehabilitation specialist can contribute significantly to improvement of patient function, to re-

Juction of risk or hazard to patients, and to enabling patients to remain as long as possible in their own familiar environment.

An understanding of the nature of the cognitive changes and their effect on patient behavior, both in general and in terms of the individual patient, is essential for interventions to be successful. The rehabilitation specialist is in a unique position to define areas of spared and impaired function, to interpret them to other members of the health team and to the family, and to modify the environment to maximize the patient's remaining abilities.

REFERENCES

1. Kramer M: The Increasing Prevalence of Mental Disorders: Implications for the Future. Read before the National Conference on the Elderly Deinstitutionalized Patient in the Community, Arlington, Va., May 28, 1981.
2. Brody EM: The formal support network: Congregate treatment settings for residents with senescent brain dysfunction. Aging 15:301–331, 1981.
3. Mace N, Rabins P: The Thirty Six Hour Day: A Family Guide to Caring For Persons with Alzheimer's Disease, Related Dementing Illnesses and Memory Loss in Later Life. Johns Hopkins University Press, Baltimore, Md., 1981.
4. Kral VA, Benign senescent forgetfulness in Alzheimer's disease: Senile dementia and related disorders. Aging 7:47–51, 1978.
5. McHugh PR: Dementia. In: Textbook of Medicine, 15th ed., ed. Beeson PB, McDermott W, Wyngaarden JB. Saunders, Philadelphia, Pa., 1976, pp 660–661.
6. Blessed G, Tomlinson BE, Roth M: The association between quantitative measures of dementia and of senile changes in the cerebral gray matter of elderly subjects. Br J Psychiatry 114:797–811, 1968.
7. Rabins PV: The prevalence of reversible dementia in a psychiatric hospital. Hosp Community Psychiatry, 32:490–492, 1981.
8. Sjorgren T, Sjorgren H, Lindgren AGH: Clinical analysis of morbus alzheimer and morbus pick. Acta Psychiatr Neurol Scand (Suppl) 82:1–152, 1952.
9. Folstein MF, McHugh PR: Dementia syndrome of depression. Aging 7:87–93, 1978.
10. Shanas E: The family as a social support system in old age, Gerontologist 19(2): 169–174, 1979.
11. Folstein M, Rabins P: Psychiatric evaluation of the elderly patient. Primary Care 6:609–620, 1979.
12. Folstein M, Folstein SE, McHugh PR: Mini-mental state: A practical method for grading the cognitive state of patients for the clinician. J Psychiatr Res 12(3):189–198, 1975.
13. Bartol MA: Nonverbal communication in patients with Alzheimer's disease. J Geriatric Nurs 5(4):21–31, 1979.
14. Goldstein K: The effect of brain damage on the personality. Psychiatry 15:245–260, 1952.
15. Rabins PR, Mace NL, Lucas MJ: The impact of dementia on the family. JAMA 248:333–335, 1982.

6 Drugs: An Obstacle to Rehabilitation of the Elderly

Dennis J. Chapron

Elderly patients seen by the physical therapist are often receiving a large number of medications, some of which are being used to improve disabilities that the therapist is treating (e.g., L-dopa for Parkinson's disease). Other drugs may be prescribed for conditions that are not of direct concern to the physical therapist yet affect the patient's response. However, regardless of a drug's indication or a therapist's professional orientation, anyone who makes a significant contribution to the care and well-being of the patient must recognize that drugs can create new illnesses or exacerbate preexisting ones.

This chapter focuses on specific drug effects that can adversely influence an elderly patient's ability to follow through on a prescribed program of physical therapy. Factors that influence drug response are discussed with particular emphasis on the aging process, and some of the common side effects of drug therapy that may present as obstacles to successful rehabilitation of the elderly patient are reviewed.

FACTORS INFLUENCING DRUG RESPONSE

The response of an individual to a medication is dependent upon both pharmacokinetic and pharmacodynamic factors. Pharmacokinetics involves how the body handles a drug, that is, it deals with the movement of drug into, around, and out of the body. Its focus is on quantitative information, such as (1) the rate and extent to which drugs are *absorbed* from sites of administration (e.g., stomach, small bowel, muscle, and skin), (2) how rapidly and extensively drugs *distribute* from the circulating blood to various sites in the body, and (3) the overall efficiency of the body's drug *elimination* processes and the relative contribution of the different systems (e.g., the kidney for urinary excretion and the liver for metabolism) that participate in the drug removal processes. Thus pharmacokinetic factors—absorption, distribution, and elimination—act in concert with the administered drug dose and govern the blood concentration of a medication.

Pharmacodynamics is the study of what a drug does to the body. It identifies the specific actions of a medication (e.g., lowered blood pressure, reduced spasticity) and examines the relationship between drug action and the amount or concentration of drug in a biologic fluid such as blood or urine. Thus pharmacokinetics and pharmacodynamics are closely interrelated and should be studied simultaneously. Since the relationship between drug concentrations in blood and drug response has been well established for numerous medications (subtherapeutic versus therapeutic versus toxic levels), the science of pharmacokinetics allows one to make good predictions of dosage requirements for an individual based on sex, age, body weight, and degree of kidney and liver function. Blood concentrations may then be used to confirm or modify initial dosage requirements.

The determinants of drug responsiveness are illustrated by a simple diagram (Figure 6-1). Drug in plasma water is accessible to its site of action. The concentration of drug in plasma water is determined by the fraction of the administered dose that is absorbed, the reversible binding to plasma proteins and tissue constituents unrelated to the site of action, and the rate of elimination from the plasma water by liver metabolism and/or renal excretion. The observed pharmacologic effect of a drug is assumed to reflect its interaction with a receptor in a target tissue. This drug–receptor complex mediates a series of biologic events that ultimately lead to a drug effect.

The magnitude of drug response is dependent on both pharmacokinetic and pharmacodynamic factors. Pharmacokinetic factors govern the concentration of drug surrounding its receptor. The concentration of drug and the affinity of the receptor for the drug determines the number of drug–receptor complexes formed. Receptor affinity and the postreceptor events may be regarded as the pharmacodynamic factors. The number of drug–receptor complexes formed often correlates closely with the magnitude of drug response. However, one must realize that the

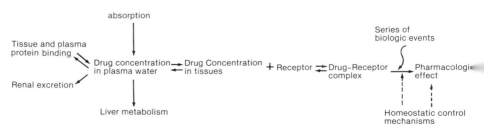

Fig. 6-1.   Determinants of drug response.

drug–receptor complex formed is often far removed from the ultimate drug effect. That is, the drug–receptor complex activates a cascade of biologic events, and the integrity of this cascade system can greatly influence drug response. Furthermore, homeostatic systems in the body will often partly counteract the drug effect, particularly during chronic drug administration.

The bulk of drug research in the elderly has been in the field of pharmacokinetics.[1,2] Many studies have shown that the elderly generally absorb drugs just as effectively as younger individuals. Age-related changes in drug distribution are very complex and difficult to interpret. However, it is clear that the decreased body weight seen in many elderly subjects should be taken into account, and dosages of medication may need to be appropriately scaled down. *Elderly patients consistently exhibit a reduced capacity for the renal elimination of drugs.* For medications that are potentially toxic and predominantly eliminated from the body via urinary excretion, the dose must be scaled down to appropriately match the degree of renal function (see Table 6-1).

The metabolism of drugs by the liver into inactive products is another critically important removal process. Studies have shown that aging seems to have a variable effect on hepatic metabolism of drugs. The metabolism of certain drugs is significantly slowed by advanced age, while others show no apparent change. Table 6-2 lists those drugs that the elderly appear to metabolize at a slower rate than younger individuals.

The study of pharmacodynamic factors of drug response in the elderly has received scant attention. There appear to be several medications that have a high incidence of side effects in the elderly that cannot be solely explained by altered

Table 6-1. Selected Drugs Removed From the Body Primarily by Renal Excretion and for Which Dosage Adjustment Should Be Considered in the Elderly

Generic Name	Brand Name
Acetohexamide	Dymelor
Allopurinol	Zyloprim
Amantadine	Symmetrel
Cephalosporins	(numerous)
Chlorpropamide	Diabinese
Cimetidine	Tagamet
Clonidine	Catapres
Digoxin	Lanoxin
Disopyramide	Norpace
Ethambutol	Myambutol
Fluorocytosine	Ancobon
Gentamicin	Garamycin
Kanamycin	Kantrex
Lithium	(numerous)
Methotrexate	(numerous)
Procainamide	Pronestyl
Streptomycin	(numerous)
Sulfonamides	(numerous)
Tetracycline	(numerous)
Tobramycin	Nebcin
Vancomycin	Vancocin

Table 6-2. Selected Drugs Metabolized at a Slower Rate in the Elderly and for Which Dosage Adjustment Should Be Considered

Generic Name	Brand Name
Chlordiazepoxide	Librium
Diazepam	Valium
Nortriptyline	Aventyl
Phenylbutazone	Butazolidin
Prazosin	Minipress
Propranolol	Inderal
Quinidine	(numerous)
Theophylline	(numerous)

pharmacokinetics. These drugs include sedatives and hypnotics, antihypertensive agents, antiparkinsonism drugs, antipsychotic and antidepressant drugs, and diuretics.

These findings of altered pharmacokinetics and probably pharmacodynamics in the elderly dictate that a special effort be made to initiate drug treatment with the lowest recommended dose and to carefully monitor response.

Many epidemiologic studies have shown that adverse drug reactions occur with a greater frequency in the elderly.[3,4] Previously discussed age-related changes in the pharmacokinetics and pharmacodynamics of drugs are partly responsible for these observations. Other factors that help to explain the increased propensity for adverse drug reactions in the elderly include the following:

1. The elderly receive more drugs than any other age group. The risk of an adverse drug reaction increases with the number of drugs prescribed.[5]

2. In the aged the presence of multiple pathologies is common. Certain disease states can influence tissue sensitivity and the pharmacokinetics of drugs (e.g., intrinsic kidney disease will decrease the contribution of urinary excretion as a route of drug elimination). Furthermore, when a drug is prescribed in a setting of multisystem disease it may exert simultaneously a beneficial effect for the condition that initiated its prescription and an adverse influence on another existing and unrelated pathology—e.g., haloperidol (Haldol), which may be indicated for psychosis, may severely exacerbate Parkinson's disease.

3. The potential for multiple medication use in the elderly is great. The incidence of drug–drug interactions can be expected to increase as additional medications are prescribed. Such interactions can result in the development of exaggerated or reduced pharmacologic responses.

Finally, a general comment on drug side effects is in order. The majority of adverse drug reactions are a direct extension of their pharmacologic effects. The physical therapist should realize that because the disposition and response to a number of drugs appears to be altered in the elderly, exaggeration of toxic drug effects at the intended site(s) of action commonly may be observed. Moreover, undesirable drug effects are often seen in tissues or organ systems other than the intended sites of therapeutic action. The present methods for delivering a drug to its intended site of action usually involve systemic administration (most commonly the oral route); thus the drugs gain access to numerous body tissues. Most medications elicit a multitude of pharmacologic actions, many of which can be deleterious to already compromised organs or organ systems. Even medications that appear to act on only one specific biologic process will often exert this action in a wide variety of tissues in a nonselective manner.

SIDE EFFECTS OF DRUGS

Selected drug side effects of concern to the physical therapist include the following:

1. Symptomatic postural hypotension;
2. Fatigue and weakness;
3. Depression and confusion;
4. Involuntary movements;
5. Dizziness and vertigo;
6. Ataxia;
7. Bladder and bowel incontinence.

It should be noted that these untoward drug effects do not necessarily occur as isolated events, but in fact often occur in clusters (e.g., fatigue, dizziness, and confusion).

Postural Hypotension

Postural hypotension (PH) is probably more common in the elderly than in any other age group. It may be asymptomatic or it may cause dizziness, lightheadedness, faintness, a feeling of weakness, or unsteadiness, or in some cases lead to syncope (a sudden but transient loss of consciousness). These symptoms appear when the patient assumes the erect posture after lying or sitting for some time, particularly in the mornings on getting out of bed. Postural hypotension may be a major cause of falls in the elderly. In the elderly population, falls are a major cause of morbidity. Falls can cause significant trauma, particularly bone fractures. In many elderly fears of repeated falls may lead to self-imposed restrictions on mobility and lifestyle. Symptoms of PH can be directly related to the sudden drop in blood pressure, which leads to a decreased perfusion of the brain and a subsequent impairment of cerebral metabolism.

When a person assumes an upright position, baroreceptor reflexes are stimulated, activating compensatory cardiovascular mechanisms that maintain blood pressure. These adaptive mechanisms are neurogenically mediated via increased sympathetic nervous system activity and include primarily reflex arteriolar constriction, reflex venous constriction, and reflex increase in heart rate so as to maintain cardiac output. There is good evidence that baroreceptor responsiveness is impaired in advanced age.[6]

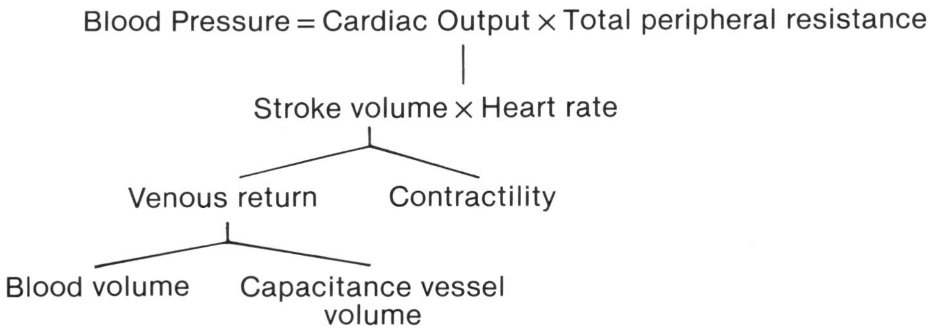

Blood Pressure = Cardiac Output × Total peripheral resistance

Stroke volume × Heart rate

Venous return   Contractility

Blood volume   Capacitance vessel
volume

Fig. 6-2.   Factors controlling blood pressure.

Figure 6-2 illustrates the many physiologic components that contribute to controlling blood pressure and demonstrates their interrelatedness. Arterial blood pressure can be expressed as the product of cardiac output and total peripheral resistance. This latter component is dependent primarily on the caliber of small vessels (mainly arterioles and to a lesser extent capillaries) and blood viscosity. Symptomatic PH leading to a reduction in cerebral perfusion may result from a decrease in cardiac output or a decrease in total peripheral resistance.

Cardiac output may be reduced by a decrease in heart rate or stroke volume. Stroke volume is largerly governed by the contractile force of the myocardium and the degree of cardiac filling. The amount of blood pumped out of the ventricles is determined by the degree of cardiac filling. The venous system contains 70 to 80 percent of the blood volume, and rapid changes in its capacitance will markedly influence the amount of blood returned to the heart. Marked reductions in either venomotor tone (leading to increased vessel volume) or blood volume (hypovolemia) will decrease cardiac filling and subsequently reduce cardiac output. Arteriolar vasodilation is the primary mechanism by which total peripheral resistance is reduced.

To establish the diagnosis of clinical PH, blood pressure should be measured when the patient is lying down, immediately on standing, and at 5 and 10 minutes thereafter. Symptoms synchronous with a fall in blood pressure of 30/20 mmHg (some authorities use 20/10 mmHg) or a systolic blood pressure falling to less than 100 mmHg should confirm the presence of clinical PH. Furthermore, remember that for patients who have low blood pressure while lying down, small postural drops may produce symptoms.

There is probably a multifactoral etiology to postural hypotension in the elderly, but often drugs may be the single most important contributing factor. Furthermore, the effects of orthostatic drops in blood pressure may be accentuated by the presence of underlying pathology (e.g., diminished cerebral perfusion from PH superimposed upon occlusive cerebrovascular disease). The risk of symptomatic PH increases with the prescription of multiple drugs, many of which may act at different or the same physiologic loci for orthostatic blood pressure regulation.

Table 6-3. Tricyclic Antidepressants

Generic Name	Brand Name
Amitriptyline	Elavil, Endep
Amoxapine	Asendin
Desipramine	Norpramin, Pertofrane
Doxepin	Adapin, Sinequan
Imipramine	Janimine, Presamine, Tofranil
Maprotiline	Ludiomil
Nortriptyline	Aventyl, Pamelor
Protriptyline	Vivactyl
Trimipramine	Surmontil

Elaborated below are the drugs I have found to be particularly important causes of postural hypotension in the elderly.

Tricyclic Antidepressants. Tricyclic antidepressants (TCAs) (Table 6-3) presumably induce orthostatic changes in blood pressure by competitively blocking sympathetically mediated vasoconstriction. Imipramine is perhaps the best studied of the TCAs. PH leading to ataxia, prolonged dizziness, and falls have been reported in approximately 20 percent of patients on imipramine.[7] Tolerance does not appear to develop to this side effect. Orthostatic blood pressure reactions can occur very early during treatment and at plasma concentrations in the subtherapeutic or low therapeutic range, suggesting that dosage reduction may not substantially alleviate symptoms. Advanced age, cardiac disease, and the presence of pretreatment postural hypotension may be important determinants to TCA-induced orthostatic drops in blood pressure. Unfortunately, little is known about the relative ranking of orthostatic potential of the various TCAs; the subject is presently under investigation.

Antipsychotic Drugs

Antipsychotic agents presumably induce their orthostatic effects by a mechanism similar to that of TCAs. There are marked differences among the specific agents regarding their propensity for inducing PH. Chlorpromazine, thioridazine, and mesoridazine have the greatest potential for inducing orthostatic changes in blood pressure. Although it is claimed that patients usually develop tolerance to the hypotensive effects of these agents, recent evidence suggests that in the elderly orthostatic effects may persist for a prolonged period.[8] Table 6-4 lists the available antipsychotic agents and ranks them according to their spectrum of common side effects. Since all these agents display similar efficacy, it seems prudent to use those with little potential for orthostatic hypotension in patients who may already present with significant postural drops in blood pressure or who have significant cardiovascular disease.

Antihypertensive Drugs. Many antihypertensive agents inhibit sympathetic neuronal function, and it is via a nonselective effect on venous and/or arterial beds that they induce orthostatic changes in blood pressure. Postural hypo-

Table 6-4. Selected Antipsychotic Drugs and Their Relative Incidence of Common Side Effects

Generic Name	Brand Name	Postural Hypotension	Parkinsonism	Sedation
Chlorpromazine	Thorazine	High	Moderate	High
Fluphenazine	Prolixin, Permitil	Minimal	High	Minimal
Haloperidol	Haldol	Minimal	High	Minimal
Loxapine	Loxitane	Minimal	High	Minimal
Mesoridiazine	Serentil	Moderate	Minimal	High
Molindone	Moban	Minimal	High	Minimal
Perphenazine	Trilafon	Minimal	High	Minimal
Thioridazine	Mellaril	Moderate	Minimal	High
Trifluoperazine	Stelezine	Minimal	High	Minimal
Thiothixene	Navane	Minimal	High	Minimal

tension is very common with guanethidine and is particularly troublesome during early treatments with prazosin. Table 6-5 lists the commonly used antihypertensive drugs and rates them according to their likelihood for inducing postural hypotension. It must be emphasized that elderly patients are often very responsive to antihypertensive agents and that inadequate baroreceptor sensitivity may make the population prone to develop significant and even disastrous episodes of postural hypotension.

Diuretics. Diuretics (Table 6-6) act on the kidney to promote salt and water loss. Overzealous use of these drugs can produce a significant reduction in the circulatory blood volume and result in decreased cardiac filling. There is no doubt that volume depletion is a major complication of diuretic treatment in the elderly.

Hypovolemia-induced orthostatic changes in blood pressure are particularly common in elderly patients taking diuretics who also have other conditions causing salt and water loss (e.g., diarrhea, vomiting, fever, loss of thirst sensation).

Nitrates. The administration of organic nitrates (Table 6-7) may sometimes lead to symptomatic postural hypotension. The sublingual route has been associated with a significant hypotensive effect, particularly when the individual is immobile and upright. These agents induce their orthostatic effects primarily via peripheral venodilatation, causing substantial venous pooling, which leads to a decrease in venous return to the heart. Nitrate-induced postural hypotension normally leads to baroreceptor-mediated reflex stimulation of heart rate and increased vascular tone. These homeostatic mechanisms help to preserve blood pressure.

Table 6-5. Commonly Used Antihypertensive Drugs and Their Relative Propensity for Causing Selective Side Effects

Generic Name	Brand Name	Postural Hypotension	Depression	Sedation
Clonidine	Catapres	Rare	Rare	Common
Guanethidine	Isemelin	Common	Absent	Absent
Hydralazine	Apresoline	Rare	Very rare	Very rare
Methyldopa	Aldomet	Occasional	Rare	Common
Prazosin	Minipress	Occasional	Very rare	Rare
Reserpine	(numerous)	Rare	Common	Common

Table 6-6. Diuretics That Can Cause Significant Salt and Water Losses and Hypokalemia

Generic Name	Brand Name
Bendroflumethiazide	Naturetin
Benzthiazide	Exna
Chlorthalidone	Hygroton
Chlorothiazide	Diuril
Cyclothiazide	Anhydron
Ethacrynic acid	Edecrin
Furosemide	Lasix
Hydrochlorothiazide	Hydrodiuril, Esidrex, Oretic
Hydroflumethiazide	Saluron
Methylclothiazide	Enduron
Metolazone	Zaroxolyn
Polythiazide	Renese
Quinethazone	Hydromox
Trichlormethiazide	Naqua

Certain drugs may significantly augment the potential for nitrate-induced hypotension. These include the following:

1. Beta-blocking agents (Table 6-8), which can depress sinus node function and result in an inadequate reflex increase in heart rate;
2. Diuretic agents (Table 6-6), which can decrease the circulating blood volume (i.e., hypovolemia) and hence potentiate the "relative" hypovolemia caused by nitrate-induced venodilation; and
3. Intake of moderate amounts of alcohol, which by itself may cause postural hypotension but which probably has an additive vasodilating effect.

Narcotic Analgesics (Opiates). Narcotic analgesics (Table 6-9) can cause significant peripheral arteriolar and venous dilatation, thus decreasing the capacity of the cardiovascular system to respond to gravitational shifts and resulting in postural hypotension. Orthostatic changes are more prominent with parenteral (intravenous, intramuscular, or subcutaneous) than with oral administration.

Vasodilator Drugs. There are numerous drugs (Table 6-10) advertised as being useful in the treatment of obstructive arterial disease. These agents are vasodilators and act by relaxing vascular smooth muscle. Interestingly, there is little evidence to suggest that any of these drugs are effective for either peripheral or cerebral vascular disease. However, these agents can cause significant postural or postexercise hypotension.

Table 6-7. Nitrates

Generic Name	Brand Name
Erythrityl tetranitrate	Cardialte
Isosorbide dinitrate[a]	Isordil, Sorbitrate
Mannitol hexanitrate	Nitranitol
Nitroglycerin[a, b]	(numerous)
Pentaerythritol tetranitrate	Peritarate, Duotrate

[a] Also available in sublingual form.
[b] Also available as an ointment.

Table 6-8. Beta-Blocking Drugs

Generic Name	Brand Name
Atenolol	Tenormin
Metoprolol	Lopressor
Nadolol	Corgard
Propranolol	Inderal
Timolol	Blocadren

Levodopa.   Chronic treatment with L-dopa frequently causes postural hypotension. This effect is believed to be both centrally and peripherally mediated. Combining levodopa with carbidopa (Sinemet) does not significantly influence the incidence of this side effect.

Continued treatment with levodopa or carbidopa is associated with a decrease in the incidence of postural hypotension. However, in many patients severe symptomatic postural hypotension may persist. This is a dose-limiting side effect, and several methods have been tried to overcome it, including elastic stockings, increased salt intake, or use of fludrocortisone (provided there are no medical contraindications).

Commentary   The physical therapist as a member of the rehabilitation team has an active role in monitoring patient response to therapeutic interventions. If postural hypotension is a presenting symptom, first evaluate the condition as it relates to activities of daily living, noting where it most frequently interferes, and then determine the cause or causes. The goal is to avoid unnecessary complications in the course of rehabilitation by assuring that pharmacologic intervention is not contributing to postural hypotension and the resulting distortion in self-care capacity.

Fatigue and Weakness

Fatigue and weakness are common complaints with the elderly and may have either physiologic or emotional etiologies. Unfortunately these complaints are often ignored by caregivers and may even be equated with poor motivation. Prolonged bed rest, muscle disuse, certain acute and chronic illnesses, and primary

Table 6-9. Narcotic Analgesics

Generic Name	Brand Name
Codeine[a]	(numerous)
Hydrocodone	Hycodan
Hydromorphone	Dilaudid
Meperidine	Demerol
Methadone	Dolophine
Morphine	—
Oxycodone[b]	Percodan
Oxymorphone	Numorphan
Pentazocine	Talwin

[a] Often marketed in combination with additional drugs.
[b] Marketed only in combination with additional drugs.

Table 6-10. Vasodilating Drugs

Generic Name	Brand Name
Cyclandelate	Cyclospasmol
Dihydrogenated ergot alkaloids	Hydergine
Ethaverine	Ethaquin, Ethatab, Laverin
Isoxsuprine	Vasodilan
Nicotinic acid	Nicobid
Nicotinyl alcohol	Roniacol
Nylidrin	Arlidin
Papaverine	Pavabid, Cerespan

depression can be obvious contributing factors. The role of drugs in producing fatigue and weakness is less well known and infrequently considered.

Beta-Blocking Drugs. These (Table 6-8) are a common source of fatigue.[9] This effect is probably due in part to their ability to reduce blood flow to muscle. With both short- and long-term treatment, heart rate is decreased at rest as well as during exercise. Stroke volume does not increase enough to compensate for the decrease in heart rate; hence cardiac output stays below pretreatment levels. During the first few weeks of treatment with beta-blockers complaints of muscle fatigue and heavy legs during and after exercise are particularly common. Although these side effects tend to disappear over time in young and middle-age subjects, little is known about the development of tolerance to these effects in the aged.

Diuretics. Diuretics (Table 6-6) may produce weakness and fatigue via several different actions. Volume depletion from excessive diuresis can decrease ventricular filling, with a consequent decrease in cardiac output, leading to decreased perfusion of muscle and producing symptoms of tiredness. Significant hypovolemia may be particularly troublesome in patients with heart failure. Increased diastolic ventricular filling is one of the necessary compensatory mechanisms that increases the force of cardiac contraction and thus helps maintain cardiac output in the failing heart.

Hypokalemia (low serum potassium) is a common side effect of diuretic use in the elderly. When the serum potassium drops below 3.0 meq/liter (particularly below 2.5 meq/liter) some degree of muscle weakness is common. The weakness is most noticeable in the legs, particularly the quadriceps muscles. In addition, hypokalemia may also produce muscle cramps and muscular pain.

Hyponatremia (low serum sodium) is a less common side effect of diuretic treatment and may produce a feeling of overall fatigue. Localized feelings of fatigue or cramps in an exercising hand or limb may also be seen. Symptoms may be seen with a serum sodium of less than 135 meq/liter but are more common when sodium levels drop to 130 meq/liter or less.

Neuropathies and Myopathies. Drug-induced peripheral neuropathies and myopathies are important but uncommon causes of weakness. Tables 6-11 and 6-12 list drugs that have been implicated in these neuromuscular disorders. The reader is referred to several excellent reviews on these topics.[10, 11]

Sedative Effects. Many drugs that have a significant sedating action may produce a feeling of weakness and fatigue. These drugs include tricyclic antidepressants (Table 6-3) antipsychotics (Table 6-4) barbiturates, benzodiazepines

Table 6-11. Selected Drugs Associated With Peripheral Neuropathies

Generic Name	Brand Name
Alcohol	(numerous)
Chlorambucil	Leukeran
Chloramphenicol	Chloromycetin
Cisplatin	Platinol
Dapsone	Avlosulfon
Disulfiram	Antabuse
Ethambutol	Myambutol
Gold salts	(numerous)
Hydralazine	Apresoline
Isoniazid	(numerous)
Metronidazole	Flagyl
Nitrofurantoin	(numerous)
Penicillamine	Cuprimine, Depen
Phenytoin	Dilantin
Procarbazine	Matulane
Vincristine	Oncovin
Vinblastine	Velban

(Table 6-13), and certain antihypertensives (methyldopa, clonidine, reserpine). Their sedative effects usually disappear after several weeks of treatment. In order to minimize the sedative potential of these drugs in the elderly, it is particularly important to begin treatment with a very low dose and increase it slowly if needed at 2- to 4-week intervals.

Finally, it should be noted that weakness and fatigue may be an early sign of a severe depressive reaction to medication. These symptoms often coexist with other signs of severe depression and include early morning awakening, appetite disturbances, and multiple bodily complaints, especially gastrointestinal.

Commentary   A patient is referred to physical therapy with the complaint of general weakness. The paramount question for the therapist (in cooperation with the other members of the rehabilitation team) is to assure that the patient has the necessary physiologic capacity to respond to treatment. Are the sodium and potassium levels appropriate? Has medication been ruled out as a contributing cause of weakness? Until satisfactory answers can be given to the questions listed, there is always the chance that the physical therapist may be attempting to treat a patient who is physiologically unable to participate in his or her present condition.

Table 6-12. Selected Drugs Associated with Myopathies

Generic Name	Brand Name
Alcohol	(numerous)
Chloroquine	(numerous)
Clofibrate	Atromid S
Corticosteroids	(numerous)
Drug-induced hypokalemia	(numerous[a])
Lithium	(numerous)
Penicillamine	Cuprimine, Depen
Procainamide	Pronestyl
Vincristine	Oncovin

[a] Primarily seen with diuretics and laxative abuse.

Table 6-13. Benzodiazepines

Generic Name	Brand Name
Alprazolam	Xanax
Chlordiazepoxide	Librium
Clorazepate	Tranxene
Diazepam	Valium
Flurazepam	Dalmane
Halazepam	Paxipam
Lorazepam	Ativan
Oxazepam	Serax
Prazepam	Verstran

Depression and Confusion

As a group, the elderly are the most susceptible to mental illness. Depression and various degrees of impairment in cognitive function are the mental disorders most commonly noted in the aged. It is particularly noteworthy that depressive reactions in the elderly often have a significant cognitive component that can easily mimic a progressive dementing process.

Drugs acting on the central nervous system (CNS) are commonly prescribed in the elderly. Their use or sudden withdrawal may precipitate significant depressive or confusional episodes in the elderly. Unfortunately, these drug reactions may not be easily recognized. Recognition of psychiatric symptoms related to drug toxicity is more difficult in the elderly than in younger patients because other or similar psychiatric problems more often may have been present prior to drug treatment.

Many centrally acting drugs have very long half-lives and with multiple dosing accumulate slowly to high levels in the body. Their adverse CNS effects develop insidiously, and there may be no obvious improvement for several days after the drug is stopped.

Sedatives, hypnotics, anticonvulsants, antipsychotics, and antidepressants can have obvious adverse effects on brain function. Less obvious, however, are the effects of drugs whose primary and intended site of action is outside the central nervous system but that because of their polypharmacologic spectrum have direct and important secondary effects on the CNS (e.g., indomethacin for arthritis, propranolol for angina).

Other drugs, via their peripheral effects, can create metabolic or cardiovascular disturbances that subsequently affect CNS function. Diuretic-induced hyponatremia or volume depletion and chronic hypoglycemia from oral antidiabetic agents are common examples of drugs indirectly disturbing CNS function and leading to confusional states. Furthermore, depression and confusion may be attributable to a prior history of poor physical and mental health, the very factors predisposing a patient to adverse CNS effects.

A previous history of depression has been shown to predispose an individual to developing severe depressive reactions to certain drugs, particularly centrally acting antihypertensive agents (e.g., reserpine, methyldopa, clonidine). It is reasonable to assume that preexisting brain damage will reduce a patient's tolerance to adverse CNS effects of drugs, confusional episodes being especially important. Finally, many metabolic, cardiovascular, and CNS disorders produce psychiatric symptoms, and great care must be taken to evaluate their contribution to the overall mental status of a patient.

In contrast to reactions related to the presence of drugs in the central nervous system, the sudden discontinuation of a drug may precipitate a withdrawal-type reaction. The onset of symptoms following sudden discontinuation of drugs is very much dependent on the individual agent involved, and onset may vary from as little as 6 hours to several days. Symptoms vary according to the drugs, but depression, confusion, and agitation are common with many withdrawal reactions.

Prevention, recognition, and treatment of drug-induced depression or confusion are of obvious importance to the physical therapist. Depressed individuals lack motivation, show disinterest, or refuse to cooperate in therapy. Even mildly confused patients may not be able to follow directions.

Because the number of drugs reported as a cause of depression or confusion is large, it is impossible to discuss each agent in this brief review. However, Tables 6-14, 6-15, and 6-16 list those drugs most commonly associated with these types of reactions in the elderly. (See Chapter 4 for discussion of detailed psychogeriatric evaluation.)

Involuntary Movements

A. Parkinsonism. Drug-induced parkinsonism is a commonly encountered clinical problem following the administration of antipsychotic medications. Symptoms usually appear during the first few weeks of treatment and are most

Table 6-14. Selected Drugs Associated With Depressive Reactions in the Elderly

Generic Name	Brand Name
Acetazolamide	Diamox
Alcohol	(numerous)
Amantadine	Symmetrel
Antipsychotic agents	(see Table 6-4)
Barbiturates	(numerous)
Benzodiazepines	(see Table 6-13)
Benztropine	Cogentin
Bromocriptine	Parlodel
Cimetidine	Tagamet
Clonidine	Catapres
Ethambutol	Myambutol
Indomethacin	Indocin
Isoniazid	(numerous)
Levodopa	(numerous)
Levodopa-carbadopa	Sinemet
Methazolamide	Neptazane
Methyldopa	Aldomet
Naproxen	Naprosyn
Prazosin	Minipress
Prednisone	(numerous)
Propranolol	Inderal
Reserpine	(numerous)

Table 6-15. Drugs Associated With Confusional Reactions in the Elderly

Generic Name	Brand Name
Amantadine	Symmetrel
Aminophylline	(numerous)
Antipsychotic agents	(see Table 6-4)
Barbiturates	(numerous)
Benzodiazepines	(see Table 6-13)
Benztropine	Cogentin
Bromocriptine	Parlodel
Cimetidine	Tagamet
Digitoxin	Crystodigin
Digoxin	Lanoxin
Indomethacin	Indocin
Isoniazid	(numerous)
Levodopa	(numerous)
Levodopa-carbidopa	Sinemet
Lithium	(numerous)
Meperidine	Demerol
Methyldopa	Aldomet
Pentazocine	Talwin
Propoxyphene	Darvon
Theophylline	(numerous)
Tricyclic antidepressants	(see Table 6-3)
Trihexyphenidyl	Artane

often observed in elderly patients. Clinically, the effect appears identical to idiopathic Parkinson's disease. Patients with drug-induced parkinsonism can show postural instability, rigidity, bradykinesia, and resting tremors. Particularly noteworthy is the nearly always *symmetrical* distribution of symptomology in the case of drug-induced parkinsonism. These untoward drug effects can create problems in sitting, in rising (from bed, chair, etc.), and in gait. There is a wide spectrum of disability associated with drug-induced parkinsonism, ranging from annoying mild tremor to severe incapacitating rigidity and bradykinesia. Certain antipsychotic drugs have a greater potential for producing parkinsonian-like symptoms

Table 6-16. Drugs Associated With Withdrawal Reactions of Which Depression or Confusion May Be an Important Component

Generic Name	Brand Name
Alcohol	(numerous)
Amphetamine	(numerous)
Anticholinergic agents[a]	Artane, Cogentin
Antipsychotic agents	(see Table 6-4)
Baclofen	Lioresal
Barbiturates	(numerous)
Benzodiazepines	(see Table 6-13)
Clonidine	Catapres
Methylphenidate	Ritalin
Narcotic analgesics	(see Table 6-9)
Phenytoin	Dilantin
Tricyclic antidepressants	(see Table 6-3)

[a] This effect is limited to agents that distribute into the brain.

than others (see Table 6-4). Thus when an antipsychotic drug is needed the selection of an agent least likely to produce parkinsonism seems particularly appropriate for those patients with preexisting disorders affecting ambulation or activities of daily living or who are already in an ongoing physical therapy/rehabilitation program.

Antipsychotic drug–induced parkinsonism can be dealt with in several ways. Symptoms, particularly when mild, usually abate within several months despite continued drug administration. The dose of antipsychotic medication may be reduced with a consequent reduction in the severity of symptoms, or one may choose to switch to another drug with a lower propensity for inducing parkinsonian reactions. Troublesome symptoms may be treated with centrally acting anticholinergic agents (typically benztropine or trihexphenidyl). These drugs are remarkably effective for relieving symptoms of antipsychotic drug-induced parkinsonism. However, it is not wise to administer anticholinergic agents with antipsychotic drugs indefinitely because of evidence suggesting that prolonged administration of this combination may substantially increase the likelihood of development of tardive dyskinesias (see below). The anticholinergic agents should be *gradually* withdrawn after about 3 months of use in order to determine if relief from drug-induced parkinsonism has occurred spontaneously. Furthermore, the elderly are especially liable to hallucinatory confusional reactions to anticholinergic drugs.

Patients with Parkinson's disease often require physical therapy. It is important to be aware that certain medications may exacerbate this disorder and/or antagonize the beneficial effects of the antiparkinsonism drugs they may be receiving. Table 6-17 lists those medications that have been reported to aggravate Parkinson's disease or block the beneficial effects of antiparkinsonism drugs.

Tardive Dyskinesias.   Tardive dyskinesias are abnormal involuntary movements occurring most often in the oral region. They are typically localized movements of the tongue, lips, and jaws, consisting of mouthing, puckering, chewing, sucking, smacking, and biting or darting movements of the tongue. Less commonly seen are choreoathetoid movements of the head, body, and limbs.

Table 6-17. Drugs That Can Aggravate Parkinsonism or Block the Beneficial Effects of Antiparkinson Drugs

Generic Name	Brand Name
Amoxepine	Asendin
Antipsychotic drugs	(see Table 6-4)
Diazepam (?)[a]	Valium
Methionine	Pedameth
Methyldopa (?)[a]	Aldomet
Metoclopramide	Reglan
Papaverine	Cerespan, Pavabid
Pyridoxine[b]	(various vitamin preparations)
Reserpine	(numerous)

[a] Further evidence for this potential adverse effect is needed.

[b] This potential adverse drug–drug interaction is seen only with levodopa and not in the combination preparation of carbidopa-levodopa (Sinemet).

Tardive dyskinesia (TD) is a late-appearing side effect of antipsychotic drug treatment. It has an insidious onset and becomes clinically evident several months after initiation of treatment. TD may appear following a reduction or withdrawal of the medication or when centrally acting anticholinergic drugs are supplemented. It is more commonly seen in the elderly, particularly females. Furthermore, in the aged symptoms are often more severe and less likely to remit following discontinuation of the antipsychotic medication. Patients with preexisting brain damage, including Alzheimer's dementia, are more likely to develop TD.

Tardive dyskinesias are typically made worse by emotional distress and are diminished or absent during sleep. Many patients are aware of their abnormal movements and may be distressed by them, particularly when they experience functional impairment, usually when their arms and legs are affected. Severe cases of TD may be complicated by difficulties of swallowing or speech, irregular respirations, and severely incapacitating movements of the axial musculature.

Levodopa and any drug with central anticholinergic action may precipitate or exacerbate this disorder.

Akathisia.   Akathisia, a syndrome of motor restlessness, is a common extrapyramidal side effect of antipsychotic drugs. It is characterized by pacing, inability to sit or stand still, continuous agitation, and restless movement and intolerance to inactivity. Akathisia is sometimes mistaken for psychotic agitation and may (inappropriately) lead to an increase in antipsychotic drug dosage. Treatment of akathisia is difficult. This side effect usually does not respond as well to centrally acting anticholinergic agents as drug-induced parkinsonism. Reduction of the dosage of the antipsychotic drug may be effective.

Essential Tremor.   Essential tremor generally involves the distal parts of the upper extremities. It may be unilateral in onset, but almost invariably it becomes bilateral and symmetrical. It is most often seen in the elderly, and in this setting it is referred to as senile tremor. Typically the tremor is decreased or absent at rest and present when the limb is held extended in a sustained posture or in active movement. It is extremely troublesome when the limb is used for tasks that require precision or careful attention, such as writing or lifting a cup or glass. This latter situation may be socially embarrassing and is often attributed to manual clumsiness. Essential tremor may be exacerbated by certain drugs, including lithium carbonate, tricyclic antidepressants, and adrenergic drugs (e.g., terbutaline). Moreover, these drugs may produce an essential tremor-like syndrome in previously unaffected individuals.

Dizziness and Vertigo

Dizziness and vertigo are important symptoms in the elderly and deserve thorough investigation. Falls secondary to these symptoms are particularly dangerous to the elderly because of their increased susceptibility to trauma, especially fractures. Furthermore, feelings of dizziness or vertigo may force individuals to severely limit their activities, leading to both social and geographic isolation.

There are a multitude of subjective symptoms that may be interpreted as dizziness. Patients may complain of a sensation of giddiness or passing out, light-

Table 6-18. Drugs That May Cause Dizziness and Vertigo by a Toxic Effect on the Vestibular System

Generic Name	Brand Name
Amikacin	Amikin
Fenoprofen	Nalfon
Gentamicin	Garamycin
Ibuprofen	Motrin
Indomethacin	Indocin
Meclofenamate	Meclomen
Naproxen	Naprosyn
Oxyphenylbutazone	Tandearil, Oxalid
Phenylbutazone	Butazolidin, Azolid
Quinidine	Quiniglute, Quinidex, Quindra
Streptomycin	(numerous)
Sulindac	Clinoril
Tobramycin	Nebcin
Tolmetin	Tolectin

headedness, floating, weakness, postural unsteadiness, or faintness. Vertigo may be thought of as a more severe form of dizziness, with a definite feeling of spinning or whirling; it is often accompanied by sweating, nausea, and vomiting.

Drugs can easily produce these types of symptoms by (1) a direct action on those areas of the brain that control motor coordination and gait, (2) upsetting brain metabolism secondary to a reduction in brain blood flow or blood glucose, or (3) a direct toxic action on the vestibular system.

Recent studies in patients over the age of 60 years have shown drugs to be a major cause of dizziness.[12, 13] Drug-induced dizziness or vertigo may occur alone or as part of a constellation of side effects.

Table 6-19. Other Drugs That May Cause Dizziness or Vertigo[a]

Generic Name	Brand Name
Acetazolamide	Diamox
Alcohol	(numerous)
Barbiturates	(numerous)
Benzodiazepines	(see Table 6-13)
Beta-adrenergic blockers	(see Table 6-8)
Cimetidine	Tagamet
Diphenhydramine	Benadryl
Hypoglycemic agents[b]	(numerous)
Isoniazid	(numerous)
Meprobamate	Equanil, Miltown
Metronidazole	Flagyl
Minocycline	Minocin
Naladixic acid	NegGram
Narcotic analgesics	(see Table 6-9)
Nitrofurantoin	Macrodantin, Furantin, Cyantin
Oxolinic acid	Utibid
Phenytoin	Dilantin
Primidone	Mysoline
Tricyclic antidepressants	(see Table 6-3)

[a] Antihypertensive drugs or other drugs capable of causing postural hypotension can precipitate these symptoms. See Table 6-5.
[b] Symptoms related to excessive reduction of blood glucose.

Table 6-20. Drugs Associated With Ataxic Reactions

Generic Name	Brand Name
Alcohol	(numerous)
Barbiturates	(numerous)
Benzodiazepines	(see Table 6-13)
Carbamazepine	Tegretol
Carbidopa-levodopa	Sinemet
Levodopa	Dopar, Larodopa, Parda
Indomethacin	Indocin
Lithium	Eskalith, Lithane
Minocycline	Minocin
Nitrofurantoin	Macrodantin, Furadantin, Cyantin
Phenytoin	Dilantin

Orthostatic hypotension leading to a decrease in blood flow to the brain is a common mechanism by which drugs cause dizziness. Every patient complaining of dizziness should be evaluated for orthostatic drops in blood pressure.

Drugs that cause dizziness and vertigo by a toxic action on the vestibular system are listed in Table 6-18. It is important to realize that certain drugs may produce irreversible injury to the vestibular apparatus (i.e., gentamicin, tobramycin, etc.), while with other drugs symptoms abate very quickly upon their discontinuation. Many drugs that have a nonselective action on the central nervous system may cause dizziness. Such drugs commonly include sedatives, hypnotics, anticonvulsants, tricyclic antidepressants, and antipsychotics. Table 6-19 lists other medications that may cause symptoms of dizziness or vertigo.

Commentary   Physical therapists treat many patients who have experienced falls. It is necessary to examine the possible role of medication-induced dizziness as a contributing cause in the accident. The ongoing presence of dizziness may require a temporary discontinuation of rehabilitation until medication adjustments can be made that allow the patient to be comfortable and motivated to participate.

Ataxia

Whereas drug-induced dizziness and vertigo create a feeling of disorientation in space, ataxic reactions to medications manifest as an impairment of upright stance and locomotion. These untoward effects are characteristic primarily of drugs that have a diffuse action on the central nervous system, and they are particularly prevalent with anticonvulsants and hypnosedatives. Of the latter, certain benzodiazepines (e.g., diazepam, chlordiazepoxide, flurazepam, clorazepate, prazepam), because of their widespread use and well-documented altered metabolism in the aged, are in my experience the most common cause of drug-induced ataxia in the elderly. These and other drugs associated with ataxic reactions are listed in Table 6-20.

Incontinence

Lack of control of bladder and bowel function is a clinical problem that can have a devastating effect on the rehabilitation effort in the elderly. Incontinence in the elderly often causes anxiety, severe distress, and depression, which can lead to so-cial isolation and can undermine the confidence and motivation essential for suc-cessful rehabilitation. The compromised bladder or bowel can be adversely af-fected by many drugs. These drugs and the complex mechanisms by which they exert their untoward effects will not be addressed in this chapter. However, when incontinence interferes with physical therapy, some simple remedies may apply. Examine the administration schedule for certain medications. For example, the administration of a rapid-acting potent diuretic [furosemide (Lasix)] minutes to a few hours prior to scheduled physical therapy for a patient with urinary inconti-nence can almost predictably lead to an unsuccessful and embarrassing session. Clearly, in patients with urinary incontinence careful attention must be paid to the scheduling of potent diuretics and physical therapy sessions. Thoughtful sche-duling of diuretic administration should produce a diuresis at a convenient time. For the patient with fecal incontinence always consider whether or not laxative use or abuse may be a contributing factor. It is not unusual for patients to experi-ence uncontrollable diarrhea the morning following a nighttime dose of a laxa-tive. Many patients with fecal soiling and urgency may benefit by the administra-tion of a rapid-acting laxative suppository [bisacodyl (Dulcolax)] an hour before a therapy session.

CONCLUSIONS

In this brief review an attempt has been made to point out to the physical thera-pist that certain drug effects can present as obstacles to successful rehabilitation. Although these deleterious drug effects can occur in any age group, the elderly are particularly vulnerable. Scheduled periodic reviews of medication use by the el-derly should include input from the physical therapist.

REFERENCES

1. Chapron D, Lawson I: Drug prescribing and the care of the elderly. In: Clinical As-pects of Aging, ed. Reichel W. Williams and Wilkins, Baltimore, 1979.
2. O'Malley K, Laher M, Cusack B, Kelly JG: Clinical pharmacology and the elderly patient. In: The Treatment of Medical Problems in the Elderly, ed. Denham MJ. Uni-versity Park Press, Baltimore, 1980.
3. Hurwitz N: Predisposing factors in adverse reactions to drugs. Br Med J 1:536, 1969.
4. Seidl LG, Thornton GF, Smith JW, Cluff L: Studies on the epidemiology of adverse drug reactions. III. Reactions in patients on a general medical service. Bull Johns Hopkins Hosp 119:299, 1966.
5. Willianson J, Chopin MJ: Adverse reactions to prescribed drugs in the elderly: A mul-ticenter investigation. Age Ageing 9:73, 1980.
6. Gribbin B, Pickering TG, Sleight P, Peto R: Effect of age and high blood pressure on baroreflex sensitivity in man. Circ Res 29:424, 1971.
7. Glassman AH, Giardina EV, Perel JM, Bigger JT, Kantor SJ, Davies M: Clinical char-acteristics of imipramine-induced orthostatic hypotension. Lancet, 2:468, 1979.

8. Branchey MH, Lee JH, Amin R, Simpson M: High and low-potency neuroleptics in elderly psychiatric patients. JAMA 239:1860, 1978.
9. Lund-Johansen P: Hemodynamic consequences of long-term beta-blocker therapy: A 5-year follow-up study of atenolol. J Cardiovasc Pharmacol 1:487, 1979.
10. Argov Z, Mastaglia FL: Drug-induced peripheral neuropathies. Br Med J 1:663, 1979.
11. Lane RJM, Mastaglia FL: Drug-induced myopathies in man. Lancet 2:562, 1978.
12. Skiendzielewski JJ, Martyak G: The weak and dizzy patient. Ann Emerg Med 9:353, 1980.
13. Blumenthal MD, Davie JW: Dizziness and falling in elderly psychiatric outpatients. Am J Psychiatry 137:203, 1980.

7 | The Aging Client and the Family Network

Carl I. Brahce

The postindustrial society of America, contrary to some popular beliefs, will need to intensify and strengthen the functions of the family as a kinship system to help elderly members live independently and with a healthy vigor for the challenges of life. The central proposition of this chapter is that the physical therapist (PT) will assume a greater responsibility for improving health care of older persons through orientation and training of the informal support system, chiefly the family network or extended kinship/social structure.

A corollary of this premise is that the family will be turning to the formal organizations providing health and medical services for assistance in caring for its elderly. Middle-aged women, who serve as the nominal caretakers of their older parents and relatives, especially will require understanding and skillful help from the entire rehabilitation team. As noted by Silverstone,[1] the informal support network for older persons goes much further than providing help and assistance; it speaks also to the affectional and social lives of the elderly, with strong implications for their emotional well-being. Sociologists and others have shown that the family network is in fact superior to the bureaucracy in performing nonuniform, nonexpert tasks like socialization and the exchange of affection in caring for older persons.[1-3] Several factors, however, are changing the intergenerational relationships of family members—more middle-aged women are engaged in careers or work, larger numbers of seniors are caring for their parents after retirement as the population of old-old persons increases, and difficulties are increasing for those elderly who do survive beyond their spouses, and even their children. One of the current problems is that American society has not yet accepted the fact that there is a rapidly increasing chronically ill aging population that will require more of a diversity of health care and supportive services in the future.[4]

The family is viewed as a resource in coping with impairment and disability, and considerable effort has been devoted to identifying the nature and extent of helping relationships.[5] Concerns about the prevalence of social isolation among the elderly are inaccurate, and it is reasonable to assume that the family network is a potential contributor to the well-being of most elderly persons.[5] In discussing the important role of family support, former Secretary of the Department of Health, Education and Welfare, Joseph A. Califano, Jr., noted that we have too often designed programs for the elderly. That is, programs that finance chronic care, for example, do little to permit and encourage home care involving the family network.[6]

The family needs to be considered as a functional unit in the delivery of health care services to the elderly. One of the major tasks of the rehabilitation team is to provide assistance to the middle-aged caregivers to facilitate performance of the nurturant role to older parents.[7] The well-being of the elderly is directly related to the extent that they receive assistance from both formal and informal support systems.[2]

The services provided by the formal support system in conjunction with those provided by the informal are important for the physical, social, and psychologic well-being of older persons. The informal support system, composed of family, friends, and neighbors, is viewed as providing the more personal and idiosyncratic services. The formal system, through voluntary agencies and large-scale governmental organizations, provides basic entitlements of health, housing, education, safety, and transportation, as well as those that are mandated under law as the Older Americans Act, Social Security, Medicare, and Medicaid.[8]

In terms of provision of care to the frail elderly, the relationship between the natural or preexisting helping network and the formal support system needs special attention. The family network may see the formal helping agency representative (e.g., the PT) as an intruder, and the professional may have difficulty in moving away from traditional service delivery techniques to work in a peer relationship in an unstructured situation. For this reason a high level of professional training and discipline is necessary to strengthen the natural system without disturbing its delicate balance.

In the following sections the preceding concepts and premises are discussed in detail. The roles and tasks of the physical therapist as a member of the rehabilitation team caring for the aged will be examined in light of changes in demographics and sociologic patterns of the aged and the family; health needs and support for elderly; the family's responsibility for care of the elderly; intergenerational relationships and caregiving; the importance of family education; and model educational strategies and programs.

THE PHYSICAL THERAPIST AND GERIATRICS

Why should the physical therapist be concerned about geriatrics? The first part of a rationale for studying geriatrics is to imply a professional requirement. As explained by Margaret Hawker in *Geriatrics for Physiotherapists,** geriatrics has fi-

---

* The reader is reminded that this work is that of an author and professional in Great Britain. Although medical practice for the elderly is emerging in the United States as an important concern of family practitioners, few medical schools offer a curriculum in geriatrics.

nally been established as a branch of general medicine concerned with the clinical, preventive, remedial, and social aspects of health and disability in the elderly.[9] The purpose of geriatric medicine, states Nichols, in the Foreword to Hawker's book, is to help restore elderly patients to activity and independence in the home setting or, if this is not practicable, to help patients gain maximum independence and live successfully in an institutional or hospital setting. As part of the total concept of reablement of elderly disabled people, physical therapy can have no meaning unless there is understanding of aging in all its implications, explains Hawker:[9]

> Without this understanding it is easy to believe that the problems of the elderly are unrewarding and insoluble—a matter for do-gooders and geriatricians. It can be more comfortable to think of people in this age group as *non-people* and so it follows that their needs and problems as individuals do not exist.

To study geriatric patients and their special needs means acknowledging that the important support usually provided the patient by the family network in the home must be assumed by the members of the rehabilitation team when the patient is institutionalized. Ideally, for any age group, but particularly the elderly, the only time that the family network should be removed or put in a position of secondary importance is in the emergency situation. As soon as the life-or-death crisis is stabilized, the family network should be invited and encouraged (through education programs and counseling as needed) to help the patient prepare for a return to the previous living environment whenever possible. If this step is not taken, the elderly patient will become dependent on the staff and make heavy emotional demands on them. Our goal is to help the family network to work with the rehabilitation team in order to meet the elderly patient's physical, psychologic, and social needs and disrupt the preexisting patterns of support as little as possible.

The physical therapist needs to recognize that aging is an evolutionary process that affects individuals at different rates and degrees and is an inescapable aspect of life, until death. Old age is not a stage like adolescence that with proper intervention the individual "gets over." It is not a phase but a culmination. The later years of life need not be filled with empty hours or days or with uselessness, but can be especially meaningful and rewarding. The older person has needs that go beyond survival or coping with the problems and losses of life—needs that enable the person to be an expressive and contributing member of the community.[10] Older persons, if they are to achieve maturity, must respond to the needs for relatedness or association with others, for creativity, for security, for individuality, for recognition, and for an intellectual frame of reference.[11]

The community is a focal point for helping the elderly remain in or regain a state of well-being in the later years. Communitywide planning must strive to meet the exceedingly complex health needs of older persons and show as great variability as in planning for child services. Convalescent facilities and rehabilitation are special problems requiring combined operations of health, welfare, and educational groups in the community.[12] As members of their society the elderly want to maintain their independence; they desire above all else to continue being active, contributing, and therefore useful members of the community in which they live.[9] The family is an important bulwark against the losses and health problems of old age. Support of the family network is now recognized as being most important for the elderly.

As the government and health care workers look for ways to provide increasingly targeted services to the elderly, one of the foci for planning is the support of the family network that gives care and assistance to elderly members.[2]

THE ELDERLY—A POPULATION IN TRANSITION

It is now accepted that increased life expectancy, the social opportunity for retirement, and independent living for older couples affects the present generation of elderly. Today's seniors, with their "on-the-go" vigor and with their general mobility despite chronic illness and sensory loss in varying degrees, would hardly be recognized as aged persons a few decades ago. They are starting new after-retirement careers, going back to college, taking part in elderhostels, being useful in volunteer activities, helping other, less fortunate elderly, assisting classroom teachers in creative teaching of elementary school children, traveling around the country and beyond in senior travel groups, assuming important advocacy roles through membership in the Gray Panthers or local organizations, and otherwise enjoying their status as senior citizens.

It has been noted that today's older citizens are contributing to a change in public attitudes or stereotypes on aging through their active roles in volunteer, advocacy, learning, and helping activities—a phenomenon never before seen in our nation, where values of youth and newness have dominated.[13] Such actions, however, do not alter the fact that many elderly, particularly those of minority populations, are still in need of medical and health care services or will be as they reach their 80s and 90s. The changing demographic patterns are in fact indicative of future health care needs of our oldest citizens, needs that will be of great economic consequence.

Since the turn of the century life expectancy has increased for the average white United States citizen from 49 to 73 years. For blacks, life expectancy at birth is lower (69 years) than it is for whites but still significantly higher than it was in 1900 (34 years). At the same time, due largely to fertility patterns, the heavy immigration from Europe in 1910 to 1920, sharply reduced mortality at birth and early childhood, and control of certain diseases, we have experienced a greater proportion of individuals living to age 65 years and older. Moreover, as today's seniors reach 65, they can now expect to live 16 more years, or until the age of 81, on the average. It is estimated by the Bureau of the Census that by the years 2010 to 2020 some 42,000,000 to 45,000,000 persons in the United States will be age 65 or older. Since the need for health and medical services rises sharply in the final decades of life, the consequence of our aging population is significant for the entire health profession.

Two results of these demographic patterns are important for the practitioner serving the elderly. First, the period in a couple's life beyond childrearing responsibility can now last for 30, 40, or more years. It is not uncommon for a retired couple to delay moving or travel after work ceases because they are caring for one or more parents.

The existence of four stages of postparental life, rather than one, have been suggested by Thompson and Streib.[14] In the first stage, *family of late maturity,* the couple's ages are generally between 45 and 54. The majority live in their own homes; 84 percent of the men and 75 percent of the women have been married. More than half of these couples still have a child under age 18 at home. The second stage is *preretirement;* chronologic ages are 55 to 64, and most such individuals are still living at home with a spouse. Sex differences in survival are apparent, with 80 percent of the men still married, compared with 62 percent of the women. One third of the still-married women continue to work. In the third stage, *the family of early retirement,* the ages are 65 to 74. Now the earlier mortality rate for men is noticeable; only 45 percent of women are married, compared to over 70 percent of the men. During the final 5 years of this period this ratio drops to 36 percent for women, and less than 10 percent of wives are still working. In the fourth stage, *late retirement,* the ages of husband and wife are 75 and above. Of men aged 75 to 79, 61 percent are still married, 49 percent at age 80 to 84, and 34 percent over age 85. The number of women still married is considerably less: at age 75 to 79 it is 25 percent; at age 80 to 84 it is 14 percent, and over age 85 it is only 6 percent. It can be seen that the health care needs of older women are related to their single status as widows or never-marrieds who often live alone. Many have outlived not only their spouses but their children as well.

A second result of demographic changes in the elderly for the health care team has to do with grandparenting. As pointed out by Troll,[15] grandparenting has become a middle-age rather than an old-age event. Earlier marriages, earlier childbirth, and longer life expectancy result in grandparents who are only in their 40s. Since these grandparents usually have only a few children, they are truly grandparents in identity and not also themselves parents of young children. In addition, owing to the increase in three- and four-generation families, the grandparent becomes a second- rather than a first-generation event (not the oldest generation). Therefore the old rocking-chair image of grandmother sitting and idly knitting or crocheting is manifestly false today. The increasing numbers of middle-aged women engaged in work careers, notes Troll,[15] have far-reaching consequences not only in adult socialization and role modeling but also in family interaction (discussed below).

THE FAMILY IN TRANSITION

For the elderly, meaningful participation in a family group is a major source of important activity.[3] Institutionalization for the elderly, whether voluntary or involuntary, is often seen as a final surrender to the realization that they can no longer care for themselves. The hope of regaining the activity level lost due to illness or natural aging processes is forever gone. Such beliefs are an important factor in postponing as long as possible the entering of homes for the aged or hospitals for the chronically ill.[3] It is for this reason that the elderly and their family network should be educated as to the importance of temporary, short-term (up to 3 months) institutional placements for rehabilitation that can or should lead to discharge to their homes (presuming that there are community/home care services to support the patient and family in the home care process—these services are currently unavailable in many areas).

The family network is important in helping the elderly to remain both active and independent. The well-being of the older person is directly related to the extent that assistance is received from both the informal support system (the family) and the formal support system (organized health and medical services).[3] The family network helping the elderly person who must deal with the bureaucracies in order to survive often serves as a mediating link between the older individual and societal institutions and organizations.[3]

Just how important is the family to the old in terms of this linkage to formal systems? In a study of informal and formal supports to maintain older people in a community, clients and their primary informal caregivers were interviewed. The research, dealing specifically with those older persons who had turned to an agency in New York City, was funded by Title III of the Older Americans Act to provide homemaker services to the marginal poor in need of such services. These services included housekeeping, shopping, and escort, as well as hands-on assistance with bathing, dressing, toileting, etc. Over half of the respondents indicated the reason for requesting homemaker services as an accident or sudden illness, while 42 percent felt they gradually needed more help in order to manage at home. Findings showed that even while formal services were being provided the family caretakers, friends, and neighbors continued to play an active role in caring for the frail elderly.[8]

The hierarchical-compensatory model shows that support-giving is generally viewed to be a function of the primary relationship of support given to the older person rather than by the nature of the task. Elderly persons, according to this concept, would prefer to receive assistance from their family. If family is not available, friends and neighbors are the next choice, followed by formal organizations.[16]

It should be emphasized that numerous studies have shown that the family remains the critical bulwark against personal and social loss for the elderly. As Sussman[3] reminds us,

> The immortal adage of "blood is thicker than water" seems to hold even in this postindustrialized period. In societies undergoing rapid changes from rural to an industrial based economy, such as Egypt, Iran, and Pakistan, family bondings are the primary structures vis-à-vis mechanisms for making bureaucracies functional and tolerable.

Lebowitz[5] elaborates on two common misconceptions about the family. The first notion concerns the low level of functional utility of the family in contemporary industrial society:

It seems common sense to many that geographic mobility, industrialization, the rise of specialized organizations for education, child care, and work have all made the family a useless or vestigial manifestation of an earlier mode of social organization. After all, the argument goes, grandparents no longer live upstairs from their married children, family gatherings rarely take place, and people would rather be in some nuclear family unit of one or perhaps two generations. Contemporary scholarship has shown this to be an inadequate conceptualization in at least two ways. First, historical studies have shown that the idealized characterization of family life in the past in both inadequate and inaccurate. Things were not so good in those good old days, as the historical and comparative studies in family structure are beginning to show. Second, the loss of family based functions has only succeeded in re-defining the notion of family into such notions as the "modified extended family" [Shanas and Streib[17] cited]. Other studies have identified the fictive kin functioning of networks of friends, neighbors, and others within a person's social environment. It is therefore safe to say that notions concerning the death of the family are misplaced and of dubious validity.

The second misconception holds that if families still function, they do not do so for the elderly. This argument says that most old people are alone, without support, and therefore both physically and socially isolated. It is true that many elderly live alone—14 percent of the men and 36 percent of the women over age 65, but it does not necessarily follow that they are isolated.[5] It has been noted that despite the geographic mobility of the United States population, many older persons who have children live close to at least one of them. In addition, such parents do see their children often.[18]

HEALTH NEEDS AND SUPPORTS FOR THE ELDERLY

The older person's family network is significant in maintaining the well-being and supporting the independent status of that individual. This informal support system becomes especially important for the chronically ill person or someone who has suffered a debilitating impairment. Such impairments, particularly progressive neurologic diseases (e.g., parkinsonism), interfere with function. As such, they threaten to undermine personal independence and those older persons need much support.[9] In addition to these illnesses, persons in the later stage of life may suffer from skeletal disorders, respiratory diseases, and sensory losses, which can be equally disabling and which often contribute to psychologic disorientation. Depression or mental impairment are especially demanding on the adult child caretakers or others in the family kinship network providing support. The physical therapist, whether involved with the patient in the home, hospital, or nursing home, can benefit from an awareness of the family role in maintaining the older patient's independence and/or facilitating rehabilitation to physical and mental capability.

To better understand the needs of older patients, let us look at normal dependencies of aging. Blenkner[19] points out that dependency for the old is a state of being, not a state of mind; a state of being in which to be old—as to be young—is to be dependent:[19]

> Such dependency is not pathological, it is not wrong; it is, in fact, a right of the old recognized by most if not all societies. It cannot be cured and the only way to forestall it is to die young.

These normal dependencies may be explained as follows:

1. Economic dependency stems from having crossed over from the productive to the consumer status in the economy. No longer a wage earner, or the spouse of a wage earner, and not having been able to accumulate sufficient savings to support oneself through 15 to 25 years of retirement, the older person typically finds himself or herself dependent on income transfers from the currently working generation, provided primarily through taxes but also by contributions from children and other younger relatives.[20]

2. Physical dependency arises from the simple fact that in the process of advanced aging muscle strength inevitably diminishes, sensory acuity decreases, reflexes are slower, coordination is poorer, and the general level of energy is lower. The ordinary chores of living—personal self-care and grooming, keeping up one's living quarters, preparing or securing food, transporting oneself from place to place, shopping, participating in social functions, etc.—become increasingly difficult, strenuous, and eventually impossible to perform entirely without aid.

3. Mental dependency arises from a decline in the power of mentation paralleling the decline in physical power, but occurring more slowly or not reaching such magnitude as to be seen as a source of dependency until quite advanced old age, and in some cases never. At that time, when deterioration or change in the central nervous system produces marked deficits in memory, orientation, comprehension, and judgment, old persons quite literally no longer can use their heads to solve their problems and direct their affairs; they must rely on the cognitive functions of others.[21]

4. Social dependency develops out of a matrix of factors and losses. As individuals age, they lose persons who are important objects and sources of affection, stimulation, and assistance. They lose roles that are the basis of status and power and avenues to social participation. They lose contemporaneity as their knowledge, values, and expectations become obsolete in a fast-changing society. They become without volition progressively isolated and disengaged nonparticipants in the surrounding social world, increasingly dependent on bureaucratized substitutes for missing kith, kin, and agents of former days, increasingly dependent on recognition by others of their rights rather that their power. They become dependent on the social conscience of the generation in positions of authority, dependent on those who currently have all that they have lost in the way of vitality and performance.[19]

* * *

Blenkner[19] suggests there are three sources of help or types of solution for the normal dependencies of aging.

The first is *self-solution,* whereby the older person seeks to modify her or his behavior or circumstances. Examples would be balancing one's budget by restricting consumption, conserving energy by restricting activities, bolstering failing memory by writing notes to oneself, countering social losses by social disengagement—a first line of defense. These methods are sensible and valid ways of coping, but they work only up to a point. The individual may increase such devices until they become pathologic and perhaps jeopardize survival of the individual.[22]

The second is the *kinship solution,* which requires the existence and proximity of children or other relatives. For those aged who are fortunate enough to have concerned and capable kin, most of their dependent needs can be and usually are met by family members providing caregiving services.

In this situation the typical old person remains in his or her own household as long as he or she is capable of personal self-care. Children or other relatives (traditionally a daughter or niece) increasingly take on or assist with the heavier tasks of housekeeping and home maintenance; provide transportation and escort; manage financial affairs; supervise health care; nurse the person in time of illness; and generally substitute their strength, mobility, and judgment for the older person's declining abilities. If or when the older person becomes too ill or frail, she or he may be taken into the caretaker's home. When the demand for intensive and skilled care rises beyond the capacity of the family network, the elderly individual may be institutionalized.

These family kinship support roles are sensible and valid, up to a point. An excessive burden of care, however, can be too much for the caretakers and other family members.[19] (Difficulties with the intergenerational aspects of caretaking are described below.)

The third solution is the *societal solution.* In this arrangement society assists its members through established programs or policies that are beyond the resources of individuals and their primary group. Examples of these solutions are social insurance, public housing and rent supplementation, and Medicaid.

It should not be thought that societal measures are adequate for health maintenance and long-term care of the elderly. There is a tremendous need to develop and expand imaginative and inventive societal solutions to the normal dependencies of aging.[19] With the extension of life after retirement and the continuing rise of inflation, many elderly are increasingly in need of a national policy of long-term care and a community care system available to all. In addition to Medicare and Medicaid, the elderly need a broad array of social and health-related services that are supportive of home-based care. The escalation of costs, coupled with a mounting public concern over the gross inadequacies of current programs, is resulting in public recognition that action is needed. An indication of this urgency is to be found in the 1981 White House Conference on Aging Act, accepting the findings by Congress that there is a great need for a more comprehensive long-term care policy (with a strong home-care component) responsive to the needs of older patients and their families.[23]

FAMILY RESPONSIBILITY IN CARE OF THE ELDERLY

Providers of health and social services to the elderly must realize that the myth of alienation of the old by the young has been found to be a groundless misconception. This social myth—that old people who live alone or apart from their children are neglected by their children—is perpetuated by aged persons themselves, especially childless old people, and by professional workers.[7,24] Elderly persons prefer to maintain their independence as long as possible, but when no longer able to manage they expect their children to assume that responsibility. Research of the past two decades shows that children give services involving physical care, shelter, and household and other related tasks, as well as sharing leisure time.[25] The family is increasingly seen as the focus for treatment in clinical or social services for the elderly.[26] A recent study showed that 87 percent of the elderly in Cleveland reported having a primary source of informal assistance available on a long-term basis, usually the family.[27] According to the National Center for Health Statistics,[28] family assistance to elderly family members comprises up to 80 percent of the care that elderly persons receive. The common forms of help are homemaker services, transportation, and personal care, including care in times of illness. As noted earlier, family members also serve as mediator and advisor to the elderly and as a linkage to formal or bureaucratic services, including health, financial, and social–recreational.[3]

The Cleveland study[27] revealed that family services are more extensive for assisting the severely impaired elderly, a fact noted by officials and gerontologists advocating policies to provide financial assistance to family caretakers. Joseph A. Califano, Jr. stated that too often programs for the elderly have been designed with the individual but not the family network in mind: "We have failed to tap the strength of the family in caring for the elderly."[6] It seems that family and kin, however defined, will continue to be those primary groups who will respond in service and kind when elderly family members call or are in need.[3]

The place of elderly in family structures is shown by studies of living arrangements of persons 65 and older. In 1970 only 4 percent of the elderly were institutionalized; the majority of senior citizens, 79 percent of the men and 59 percent of the women, lived in family situations, and most resided in their own homes.[29] Since women live longer than men and have thus less choice in partners for second marriages, they are more active in linkage activities within the family.[3] Age and number of children seem to be the most important predictors of moving into a family member's household when living alone becomes untenable because of diminished health and mobility.[3]

Four kinds of relationships or dimensions have been suggested to assess family or kin structure:[15] (1) residential proximity—how close relatives live to each other; (2) interaction frequency—how often relatives visit, phone, or write each other; (3) economic interdependence or mutual aid; and (4) a variety of more subtle qualitative measures, such as the valuing of "familism," the transmission of values, and the strength of affectional bonds.

Researchers agree that the kinship ties are strongest between female members in the helping relationships. It is usually the daughter or daughter-in-law who act as caretaker. The mother–daughter relationship tends to be stronger than the mother–son bond from adulthood on. Other researchers have found that the sister–sister tie is stronger than either the sister–brother or the brother–brother tie). Although most studies show a bias toward female-linked relationships in the family network (residence is closer to wife's parents; interaction is greater with wife's relatives, is mutual and more frequent along female lines; and affection is said to be greater among women), Adams found little sex differentiation in his research on kinship interrelationships except for patterns of mutual aid. More men than women gave help in both money and services, such as work in the house, to their parents. Also, since women outlive men in the later years of life, more older men than women actually live in families. Widowers are much more likely to remarry than widows. On the other hand, older widows (closer to their daughters) are more likely to move in with children, usually daughters, when they no longer can manage to live alone than are older widowers.[15,30,31]

As pointed out earlier, the current generation of elderly are a hardy cohort, and research of the past several years shows that they prefer to live independently in their own household. Even after a spouse dies, and faced with the emotional difficulties associated with bereavement, older persons strive to maintain their independence. The important fact for PTs and others on the health care team to recognize is that the family members do provide meaningful strength and support to the elderly across many dimensions.[3,30] As Sussman states,[3]

> The continued psychological well-being of the aged, similar to the needs of persons at all stages of life, is largely dependent upon a high level of activity, involvement with other persons, and with interests beyond their own personal lives. Meaningful participation in a family group is a major source of such activity for the elderly.

INTERGENERATIONAL RELATIONSHIPS AND CAREGIVING

Research in intergenerational relations is a relatively recent phenomenon. As observed by Troll,[15] there is nearly a 30-year gap between parent–child relationships dealing in the launching stage, when the parents are in early middle age, and relationships involving aged parents and their adult children. Between these two points both parental and child couples are growing older, but there are few data on life-cycle patterns of behavior in this period.

During the first phase, middle-aged parents are frequently visited by children, and parents provide help to children in the form of services or money. The American norm requires independence of the newly married couple. They are expected to establish a home separate from both sets of parents, raise their children, and be economically independent, by virtue primarily of their own efforts and successes. At the other end of the age scale the stereotype of old parents is that they desire dependence on their adult children and demand services, moving in with children where possible, but generally neglected and unwanted.

Actually, most young couples in the United States seem to live reasonably close to both sets of parents, receive help in the form of either services (babysitting) or money, and visit often. Most old parents prefer to live alone and to see their children frequently. Blenkner[7] has described the concept of "filial maturity" for that stage seen as part of the developmental sequence representing the healthy transition from genital maturity to old age. This concept has its own sequence of stages. A filial crisis may be said to occur in most persons in their 40s or 50s, when the individual's parents can no longer be looked to as a rock of support in times of emotional trouble or economic stress but may themselves need their children's comfort and support. Successful accomplishment of the filial task or performance of the filial role promotes filial maturity. This has its own gratification, leading into and preparing the middle-aged person for successful accomplishments of the developmental tasks of old age—the last of which is to die.[7]

In this concept Blenkner refutes the earlier concept of role reversal formerly held by many gerontologists—that as the parents age they take on the child's former dependent role while the child assumes the parents' supportive role. Blenkner postulates that the son or daughter does not assume the parental role toward the parents but rather grows into a mature filial role. This role is that of being depended on and therefore means being dependable. In achieving this filial maturity that occurs in middle age, the adult turns again to the parent, no longer as a child but as a mature adult with a new role and a different love. The adult child sees the parents for the first time as individuals with their own rights, needs, limitations, and life histories that to a large extent made them the people they are long before the child existed. As Blenkner explains, this is what parents want of their children; this is what society expects; this is what many Americans do accomplish, with varying degrees of success, in their late 40s and 50s. It is also one of the ways in which the adult children prepare themselves for their own aging, through identification with the parent, just as in childhood they similarly prepared for adulthood.[7]

One of the major roles of the therapeutic professions can be that of helping the middle-aged family member, client, or patient accomplish this task as best as possible. This is important because it will ultimately determine how successfully the challenge of growing old is met.[7]

The importance of reciprocity in this relationship is suggested by Troll.[15] The significance of the parent–child relationship is that it continues throughout life. Parents who continue to mature throughout their lives, who accept their own development as meaningful and satisfying, are really assisting their children to mature in turn.

The situation of the caretaker as helper to elderly parent(s) or relatives—i.e., one who carries out the concept of filial maturity and is responsible—can become critical for the middle-aged caretaker. Usually a woman whose children have just left the home nest may be in the process of adjusting to important changes in her own life cycle. These changes for the middle-aged woman may have to do with conflicting obligations to teenaged children or to spouse, the postponement of assuming a career again, or returning to school to learn new skills. Since members of the older generation are remaining independent longer, the adult caretaker may also be coping with retirement. There are many parent–child pairs in which the children themselves are at or near retirement.[32] In addition to these pressures, career obligations may conflict with the caregiving role, especially with the increase in numbers of women now in the labor force. This middle-age crunch of responsibility is a time of midlife crisis for the adult caretaker; she becomes the sandwiched generation.[33]

As illustrated earlier, certain differences between the age cohorts of adult children and aged parents are a result of both social changes and personal expectations due to changes in the life cycle. In the matter of providing supports these two generations may experience difficulty or conflict. The first fact to be considered is that for middle-aged and older parents, or young-old and very old generations, parents and children are adults or social equals. The earlier socially sanctioned power imbalance based on the minority position of the child and the child's economic dependence is gone. Also gone, along with the public entitlements of social insurance, social security, and Medicare, is the reverse situation—complete economic dependence of an elderly parent on children. Along with this status, both older generations, if still married, retain primary emotional investments in and obligations to their marriage partners. (This becomes more complicated in the case of in-laws.[34])

Second, regardless of time or social context, members of different generations have vastly different life experiences and are products of different social influences. In this sense the middle-aged and old will continue to bring different motivations, aspirations, beliefs, and expectations, as well as different capacities, to their mutual relationships. Even when they may experience the same historical event, such as war or depression, their different age locations and cohort memberships means the event will have varying impacts on their lives. Each has encountered unique life situations, and "consequently, the middle-aged and old have self-interests that are potentially productive of conflict in the societal arena—and of strain in the intergenerational relationship."[34]

The intergenerational difficulties may be of two orders: those arising from age structure alone, and those compounded by longstanding conflict within the family.[32] The first group is marked by the following:

1. The problem of fatigue. Pressures on the caretaker may be too much, particularly in the case of illness or incapacitation.
2. The problem of competing demands. Particularly pressured are those sons or daughters caught between spouse, children, and the elderly parent.[32]

Intergenerational difficulties created by old patterns of conflict within the family include the following:[32]

1. The problem of anaclitic rage and depression. Adults may be unable to accept a dominant parent's decline.

2.   The problem of the wrong survivor. If the family script has called for the other parent to die first, it may be hard for members to relate to the real survivor.

3.   The problem of sibling rivalry. Sibling rivalry may persist to the very deathbed of the courted parent. Generally, one sister or brother is doing most of the work; another appears to be getting most of the credit. Often the put-upon sibling is not giving the other a chance to do a fair share because the purpose is to show how unworthy the rival is. None of this is helped by a parent who instinctively grasps the benefits to be derived from the competition.

4.   The problem of the unemancipated son or daughter. Most adolescents separate painfully from their childhood selves with all their dependence on parental approval and all their fantasies of parental omnipotence, but a few adults continue to behave as if governed by an ambivalent drive for independence. Sometimes the aging adolescent foregoes marriage and remains an uneasy son or daughter in the home. If the parent is unable to let go, the relationship may be marked by alternate periods of appeasement and explosion.

These problems can be synergistic, but generally several approaches can be useful. The following are applicable:[32]

1.   Encouraging all parties to make reasonable demands before these take the form of confrontation improves the climate.

2.   Emphasizing that *now* is not *then* improves reality testing, even without much insight or working through.

3.   Accepting the negative part of the ambivalence and putting it in the context of the total behavior promotes better relations.

4.   Redefining the old person as interactive reduces guilt and restores perspective. This is especially important if the parent is becoming confused or going into an institutional placement.

One of the common errors of adult children is to exclude the parent from planning or decision-making on the grounds that they are too fierce to be faced, too impotent to be counted, or too vulnerable to be told. In so doing, the adult children reduce the older parent or relative to objects. Similarly, children caretakers need to understand that confusion is not constant and that even persons incapable of ultimate responsibility may contribute to a decision. Persons not fully oriented may still be aware of their own feelings and sensitive to the way others in the family are responding to them.

THE IMPERATIVE OF EDUCATION FOR FAMILY CARETAKERS AND PROFESSIONALS

The beneficial aspects of caretaking within the family are strengthened with an educational intervention offering both knowledge and emotional support to caretakers.[35] Professionals and social workers providing health and medical services to elderly patients could similarly profit from an opportunity to learn about the realities of the aging process and the pitfalls or stress points in the vital function of family care of the elderly.[36] Lebowitz noted that most older persons are tied into a network of social support (primarily adult children) and that fictive kin (friends and neighbors) provides important supportive services, and identified certain gaps in research findings that need attention. One fundamental gap in knowledge concerns the manner in which portions of support systems are activated in order to provide assistance to the older person:[5]

> We do not have the basic understanding of the decision [making] process whereby an older person reaches out for help or in which family members or friends offer support. Our studies have not captured the complexity of this dynamic situation.

Research also has failed to conceptualize adequately the dynamic processes of identification, conflict, evaluation, and decision that are characteristic of the relationship between family members. Too little is known about disagreements between older people and their family or friends, or the dimensions of depression. Someone who is depressed is unlikely to seek help and often is reluctant to accept it when offered. Consequently, supports may not be activated. This issue represents another gap in knowledge.[5]

Institutionalization of the elderly is not required for the majority of aged persons. In maintaining the psychologic well-being of the elderly family member the family plays a critical role; the health care professional can be a consultant in the helping pattern of services. To the aged, institutionalization, as suggested previously, may be seen as a final surrender of self-care and meaningful activity. One recommendation to improve hospital rehabilitation is to increase the flexibility of hospital rehabilitation programs sufficiently to allow the elderly person to return to the community as quickly as possible[3] (e.g., short home visits during the rehabilitation process).

Nothing is more unbearable to the older person than being alone and feeling unwanted. The family has the capacity to give the older person a sense of being accepted and being loved. When the family can give its love and understanding the physical handicaps that older persons must live with become easier to bear.[4] It is therefore necessary to support the patient–family contact during institutional-based rehabilitation so as not to alienate the patient from the family network in the name of rehabilitation. In home-based rehabilitation programs or institutional-based programs with a strong family education and counseling component both the patient and the family are more likely to be accepting of the final outcomes.

Butler[37] has pointed out that countertransference in the classic sense occurs when mental health personnel find themselves perceiving and reacting to older persons in ways that are inappropriate and reminiscent of earlier patterns of relating to parents, siblings, and such key childhood figures. Since the professional relationships are critical for physical therapists as well as professionals involved in psychotherapy, difficulties from ageist attitudes of staff are worth noting. Butler states that staff members have to deal with leftover feelings from their personal pasts that may interfere with their perceptions of an older person. They also must be aware of a multitude of negative cultural attitudes toward the elderly that pervade social institutions as well as individual psyches. The GAP Report, *The Aged and Community Mental Health, 1971,* listed the following major reasons for negative attitudes of staff toward treating older persons.[37]

1.   The aged stimulate the therapist's fears about his or her own age.
2.   The aged arouse the therapist's conflicts about her or his relationship with parental figures.
3.   The therapist believes that he or she has nothing useful to offer older people because she or he believes that they cannot change their behavior or that their problems are all due to untreatable organic brain diseases.
4.   The therapist believes that psychodynamic skills will be wasted in working with the aged, since they are near death and not really deserving of attention.
5.   The aged patient might die while in treatment, which could challenge the therapist's sense of importance.
6.   The therapist's colleagues may be contemptuous of efforts on behalf of aged patients. (One often hears the remark that gerontologists or geriatric specialists have a morbid preoccupation with death; their interest in the elderly is therefore "sick" or suspect.)

Another difficulty that may affect the health care worker's treatment of the aged is what seems to be a human propensity for hostility toward handicapped individuals, stemming from unconscious overidentification with older persons, especially those who are physically handicapped or thought to be crippled and powerless. What may result is oversympathetic concern, resulting in hostility.[37]

On the whole, we do not know much specifically about old age, since most clinical experience and research has been of the sick and institutionalized rather than the healthy, active elderly. One consequence of this limitation, observes Butler,[37] is the loss of the more enduring, intensive relationship of treatment for personnel and patients, which could be an important source of data about older persons as well as a check on therapist evaluation of them.

Similarly, the physician rarely encounters a member of the older patient's family (except the spouse) until the patient's capability for living independently is challenged.[26] At the point where the elderly patient's functional independence is challenged, the physician must be aware of potential family problems and strengths that relate to the elderly patient's care.

As noted earlier, adult caretakers may be facing crises of their own when their parents become dependent or disabled. In review, these could include loneliness secondary to the children leaving home (that is, the empty-nest syndrome); the necessity of reexamining personal relationships with spouse and children; conflict with other siblings over the caretaking responsibilities; a renewal of earlier communication or interrelationship conflicts between themselves and the parent; facing one's own middle-life adjustment problems, including one's own aging. In addition, a problem that is sure to be exacerbated in the future is that of the woman caretaker being forced to delay or interrupt her own activities and priorities (education or career).

The supportive role for the therapist is emphasized by Milloy.[38] In this perspective the worker's interest should center on helping the older person maintain external and internal depleting and restorative forces—the nature of the ego and its capacity to deal with both internal and external stress. The worker's proper concern, then, is not so much pathology and treatment as those ego and life forces that are still intact or capable of restoration. The worker should acquire a *longitudinal view* of the client in order to determine the strength of the client's anchorages, how well they have served the client, and how adequate they are in the present. This perspective means viewing aging as a developmental stage in order to evaluate both the older person's success in mastering the tasks and crises of previous stages as well as the residue of unsolved problems complicating the mastery of current crisis.[38] The professional therefore requires a knowledge of the aging process from a psychologic perspective, including the patient's history of ego functioning at various age levels. The worker also should be familiar with the degree of conflict that might exist between the client's and society's expectations with regard to client role performance in various statuses, including spouse, parent, child, older person, unemployed person, and roles in relation to race, religion, education, and occupation.

It is important to realize that the transition from one set of roles to the other cannot be accomplished without great pain and anxiety, not only for the older person but also for those who are affected by role definition or participation in roles, such as adult children when they feel they should assume roles of parents to their own parents.[38]

The older person's losses may also stem from the painful loss of spouse; the necessity of giving up a lifelong occupation or career because of illness; or simply the loss of health. Coping with bereavement can be important in maintaining the older person's sense of purpose or value in living. Such adjustment may be expressed in depressive reaction. The older client may seem to have lost an anchor, a habit pattern of daily living related to the lost person. Although the patient may appear not quite oriented, she or he will not have lost touch with reality. But reassurance is needed, expressions of interest from intimate persons, help in making new connections and activities. The point is that the health care therapist must make an unusually heavy emotional investment in the older client, not a personal one, but a professional one, through which the client learns that his or her own thoughts and feelings are truly important.[38]

As noted earlier, an overinvestment in the older client to satisfy the therapist's own needs is not beneficial. Rather, the therapist needs to have a controlled empathy with the client that is focused to help the client.

A knowledge of available community resources can be useful for the health care worker in assisting the family. The two most important criteria[38] for utilizing any services are as follows: (1) Will using the service increase or maintain the client's capacity for self-directed behavior? (2) Will it tend to lessen the client's sense of isolation and increase the feeling of being needed?

The PT may find it necessary to assist the family in decisions about living arrangements or resorting to institutionalization as the condition of the patient worsens. In answering questions such as the need for institutional care, the PT needs to be cognizant that each person is a product of unique life experiences. Plans for living arrangements should be based on the principle that *as long as a person gains more gratification than pain from living in the community, it is better to help the patient remain there.*[38]

The adult child who seeks assistance in relation to caring for an aging parent or relative can be helped in several ways. One of the most important is in separating reality from the mass of feelings that color it:[38]

> The worker can be most supportive if he [sic] can help the client understand that his parent is not a child for whom he must assume complete responsibility: the parent is an adult, who, although suffering from serious limitations, has a right to make decisions and to take responsibility for the consequences of those decisions.

Specific programs that have been developed to assist elderly in coping with losses and provide support for family members are discussed below.

FOUR CONCEPTS—EDUCATION STRATEGIES TO SUPPORT THE AGING CLIENT AND THEIR FAMILY NETWORK

A perspective is emerging that the practicing PT will ultimately be involved with families providing assistance to their elderly. In such involvement the professional can benefit from an understanding and from knowledge that goes beyond the functions of technical competence and practical skills. In order to illuminate some new dimensions with regard to family caretaking I will describe four programs that I consider to be innovative, relative, and timely. The descriptions cover the reason or rationale and purpose of the programs, clientele served and family relationships, program objectives, program content, and results, with implications discussed in subsequent sections. I hope that the PT will gain a clearer understanding of the scope of the problem as well as the opportunities involved in approaches to care of the elderly that involve the family network as a part of the rehabilitation team.

Peer Supports for Older Adults

The Peer Support System was started in 1978 as part of the psychosocial component of the Turner Geriatric Clinic, an outpatient clinic at The University of Michigan Hospital, Ann Arbor. It began as a program of monthly health education workshops planned and implemented by a group of peer counselors—that is, older persons. As of September 1980, 48 older men and women had been trained as peer counselors, and approximately 2500 persons had participated in some phase of the program.[39]

The staff at Turner Clinic were struck by the need for information and attention of the older persons who came as patients. Frequently they would tell the staff of their frustration with doctors who only had a few minutes to give to each patient, "rushing me in and out," or the family doctor who said, "What can you expect, you're just getting older. Nothing can be done about it." Despite relatively good health, many of the older persons had generalized worries about the future and a set of specific concerns (e.g., treatment of chronic conditions, exercise, diet, and the effects of new drugs and their interaction with drugs already taken). Part of their worries, the staff noted, were a result of too much rather than too little information from the mass media. The staff realized that many of their patients' concerns were shared by many—e.g., worries about cataract operations, memory lapses, hearing loss, stiffening joints, and general uncertainties about how all of these might threaten their independence. Once a program to address this need was decided upon, the staff agreed that they needed input from the elderly before drafting the program.

The first step was to identify a nucleus of older adults (from patients) who had leadership potential and who might be willing to serve as peer counselors. Patients, colleagues, and social agency staff were asked to suggest candidates. Subsequently, 12 persons became the first peer counselors. It was subsequently decided by counselors and staff to organize a series of workshops. A list was compiled for early participants to select topics of interest for future workshops.

An evaluation form was composed for participants to complete after each workshop. Peer counselors prepared and distributed a flyer and sent publicity releases to the local newspapers and radio stations. Arrangements were made for cooperation with the Washtenaw County Council on Aging. Small group discussions were role-played so that peer counselors could practice leading a group.

The first workshop attracted 60 persons, even though it snowed that day. The eagerness of the older persons to participate and contribute was noted. Audience members shared information on funerals, bad insurance companies, and problems in returning purchases to stores, along with evidence of discrimination against the elderly consumer.

The program objectives and methods are shown in Table 7-1.

The peer counselors represented a wide range of backgrounds and personalities: 12 were male, 36 female; ages ranged from 52 to 83 (the 52-year-old faced early retirement due to disability; next youngest was 60), with an average age of 70; 2 were single, 21 married, 23 widowed, and 2 divorced; 9 had completed elementary school, 4 had some high school, 13 had some college, and 13 had a college degree.

A peer counselor who is legally blind helped organize the Low Vision group and workshop. She later counseled individuals personally as well as low-vision clients over the telephone. She has since organized an Eye Information Center, talking to people on a drop-in basis. Not all who started counseling continued; some found it upsetting, time-consuming, or "not for them." When a peer coun-

Table 7-1. Program Objectives and Methods

Objectives	Methods
1. To provide up-to-date information on issues affecting the health and well-being of older people	Speakers at monthly workshops Handouts and brochures at workshops Once-a-month peer counselor in-service training meetings Development of informational materials, e.g., Housing Booklet
2. To involve older people in the planning and implementation of the program	Peer counselor group Short evaluations at each workshop Long checklist of topics distributed to workshop participants at regular intervals Telephone evaluations at Turner Clinic and other sites
3. To reach a large number of people with differing needs	Expansion to three new sites Wide publicity in senior newsletters, church bulletins, newspapers, and radio Peer counselor talks in senior housing, churches, and senior centers Peer counselor home visits Wide range of small groups and workshop followup sessions
4. To provide varying levels of involvement, various levels of entry	Encouragement of referrals from inpatient and outpatient social workers in medical and psychiatric divisions; provision of program information to hospital discharge planners and social agency personnel; range of services from large monthly workshops through one-to-one counseling at home Small groups directed to specific targets— e.g., to those with severe memory loss or hearing or visual impairment, exercise Clinic staff informed of programs; provision for peer counselor, student, and/or project staff involvement with clients having psychosocial problems, i.e., loneliness, isolation, lack of mobility
5. To provide a link with community resources	The best speakers on each topic Time for questions and individual discussions with speakers Availability of literature on what agencies in the area offer services pertinent to the topic discussed Peer counselors informed of resources and changes in personnel and locations to pass on to workshop participants, clients, and group members Special forums on timely issues, e.g., transportation workshop when Senior Dial-A-Ride schedule changes were made; elderhostel information meeting, where people who had been to elderhostel spoke and registration information was distributed

selor was appropriately matched with a client and was given staff support and suggestions, the result was valuable for both persons.

Frequently, workshops served to introduce new ideas and to stimulate interest in pursuing a subject in more depth. As a result, the formation of small groups grew out of workshop presentations.

Although few peer counselors would have called themselves advocates, the fact that they were better informed about services and resources than the average person and had a number of channels through which to spread information placed them in this role. One peer counselor was particularly effective in convincing persons that they have the right to ask questions and receive answers from ophthalmologists and others who work with the visually impaired. Others have written letters to editors and taken part in community planning meetings and advisory groups. Most important, according to the Turner Clinic staff, they are models, by their behavior and attitudes, for older adults who are active participants in their community and able to take responsibility for issues affecting their interests and the needs of those less able. One visitor remarked to a group, "I just can't wait to get old."[39]

Older Women Caring for Disabled Spouses

A multiservice program directed toward women who are caregivers of their elderly spouses evolved into a respite project that incorporated several community-based supportive services. The original impetus for the wives' support group started in Marin County, California in 1977. The initiator was a woman who had cared for a stroke-disabled husband for 17 years and who also was a leading advocate for the development of a community day care program.[40]

The project funding initially received came from the Senior Community Employment Program (Title V, Older Americans Act). Primary outreach efforts were directed toward the day care population, where the number of women involved in caregiving was significant. Of the participants 50 percent were men, and 85 percent of them were cared for by their wives. This was comparable to research findings that men are more likely than women to be cared for by a spouse. Such women are identified in the literature as being "the hidden victims," a high-risk group of elderly women. For such caregivers the emotional strain and the physical demands of caregiving are superimposed on the stress they already are experiencing in attempting to cope with their own aging processes. Most of the women experience isolation, loneliness, and role overload.[40]

The primary purpose of the wives' group was to build mutual support. They began with monthly meetings, but these were expanded to twice monthly because the caregiving wives wanted more time for educational programs. For these sessions resource persons were invited to address issues of concern that ranged from preparing financially for a spouse's institutional care to the physiologic and psychologic aftereffects of a stroke. All meetings took place at the day center, with arrangements made for the husband to attend the center that day if he was not a regular participant. Group meetings were facilitated by coleaders, the group's founder, and a social worker who also served as program director at the day center. Their role was to encourage each woman participant to express her feelings and to foster a nonjudgmental atmosphere where others refrained from giving advice.

As with similar groups, the participants were experiencing stress and a prevailing sense of isolation, both social and emotional. The majority of women were caring for husbands who were brain-injured to some degree. Since many of the spouses no longer had full capacity for empathy or interpersonal sensitivity, they could rarely satisfy their spouses' needs. The group's founder described this as a loss of closeness, of loving. The group experience gave the wives an opportunity to share common experiences as well as to explore alternative methods of coping and problem solving.

One general need surfaced—the need for adequate, affordable respite services in the community that would relieve the women of daily demands of caregiving. Most of the women could not afford the community's proprietary (for profit) home care services. This issue led to the submission of a grant proposal to a local foundation to support a 2-year respite care service. The Respite Project was funded in June 1979 for 2 years. The $40,000 grant provided for three main program elements: home care, overnight respite, and community/professional education.

The overall objectives of the Respite Project were as follows:

1.   To provide immediate respite for the wives and relieve their financial concerns by offering a few hours of home care each week and an extended out-of-home respite session at no cost; and

2.   To develop and publicize the issue of older women as wives and adult caregivers and the special problems they face.

The project also was designed to demonstrate the benefits of a coordinated system of support services. The group was considered to be an integral part of that system. The Project provided funding for one full-time nurse whose time was divided each week among the 12 to 15 wives requesting this service. The extent of this service was limited to about 4 hours a week per couple. Combined with day care, however, the service expanded the respite available to the women, while giving them the assistance they needed in the home. The nurse's role included assisting with household tasks, shopping, meal preparation, and other tasks with which the couple needed assistance. An extra advantage to the women that the nurse provided was not anticipated—added emotional support. The dependability and continuity of this support as well as the familiarity that developed between the wives and the nurse proved to be important elements of care that could not have been provided if the wives had had to depend on the sporadic availability of home help from other agencies.

One benefit was that the respite service provided both husband and wife the opportunity for periods away from the intense interaction and stresses inherent in their relationship. It had been 3 to 12 years since any of the wives had had a vacation. All commented on the peace, quiet, and rest they were able to enjoy. Comments on the benefits ranged from, "The nurse's visits raise his mood," to

"One day away from me—he would have to enjoy the change." The reactions demonstrated the positive effects of the respite program for the husbands as well as the wives. Two special programs were generated in the Project: (1) a community workshop was directed to both the public and health care providers (the latter generally fail to understand the ongoing problems faced by wives once the husband is discharged from the acute care or rehabilitation facility); (2) a videotape was produced with the help of a nonprofit agency in the community—entitled "Women Who Care: Living with Disabled Husbands," the videotape focuses on one of the couples involved in the Project. Personal interviews with other participants provided information on their personal experiences. The community workshop attracted many women and other family caregivers as well as health care providers.

The Natural Supports Program (New York)

The purpose of Natural Supports Program (NSP) was to explore the nature and extent of care provided by families to the aging and to determine how services might be designed to enhance and prolong caregiving efforts.[41] NSP was initiated in October 1976 by the Community Service Society of New York based on the premise that a family's caregiving efforts on behalf of its elderly can be supported by the development of services designed specifically for its members. NSP has concentrated on the role of the family, both nuclear and extended. The Project sought to supplement rather than substitute for the care provided by informal supports.

Two distinct service modalities were utilized: (1) family-centered social casework, and (2) community based group services.

Objectives of NSP were as follows:

1. To promote and document the development and use of groups comprised of caring relatives of the aging in order to strengthen their caregiving capacity;
2. To develop a variety of community-based group models and assess their replication potential across a diversity of family types and communities; and
3. To provide training for group leadership and to attempt to mobilize or develop community organizational structures that will provide for local accountability and maintenance of these groups.

Four contrasting areas of New York City were chosen to assess the applicability of service models in relation to a variety of community and population characteristics. The areas varied in demographic characteristics, types of family constellations, extent and nature of services for the elderly, and geographic proximity of the older person to supports.

Community assessment meetings for caregivers that also involved professionals from related agencies were held. Information on the aging process, nature of the caregiving role, and services–benefits for the elderly was provided by speakers, resource persons, demonstrations, and literature. Supportive services were offered in small discussion groups comprised of up to 12 caregivers, a leader, resource person, and a recorder. They provided an opportunity for ventilation of concerns, problem solving, and service requests. A social worker was present at each program to deal with crises and individual service requests.

The age breakdown of attendees ($n = 266$) indicated that 18 percent were between 29 and 39 years, 54 percent between 40 and 59 years, and 19 percent above 60 years old (9 percent no response). The racial composition was of 80 percent white, 10 percent black, and 10 percent other. The religious affiliations were 28 percent Catholic, 27 percent Protestant, 32 percent Jewish, and 4 percent other (9 percent no response). Income distribution indicated that 30 percent had an annual family income exceeding $20,000, 20 percent between $15,000 and $20,000, 18 percent between $10,000 and $15,000, 17 percent between $5000 and $10,000, and 11 percent reported a family yearly income below $5000. Marital status indicated that 44 percent of the attendees were married, and 24 percent were single; an additional 15 percent were either separated, widowed, or divorced (17 percent did not respond).

Attendees indicated the following breakdown of ages of the older person of concern ($n = 175$): 14 percent were between 60 and 69 years, and 86 percent were above 70 years of age. Income distribution included ($n = 88$) 41 percent receiving less than $3000 per year, 34 percent between $3000 and $5000, 13 percent between $5000 and $10,000 and 6 percent had yearly incomes above $10,000 per year. Six percent ($n = 38$) were receiving Supplemental Security Income and 20 percent Social Security. The marital status ($n = 100$) indicated that 66 percent were widowed, 21 percent married, 5 percent single, and 7 percent divorced. As to living arrangements ($n = 229$), 37 percent of the older relatives were living alone, 55 percent were living with either a spouse or the attendee, and 8 percent were institutionalized.

Attendees reported disabilities of 187 older relatives of concern as follows: 59 percent had multiple disabilities, with 35 percent reported as confusion, 35 percent depression, 34 percent mobility, 26 percent vision, 19 percent hearing, 16 percent heart condition, 10 percent for each use of hand/arms and for speech, and 9 percent for bowel and bladder control. Attendees were asked to check the number of formal services received by their older relatives. Of 72 responses, 69 percent were not receiving any formal services and 30 percent were receiving one or more services. Of the attendees ($n = 200$), 60 percent reported that they were the only caregiver for their older relative; 21 percent reported one other person involved, and 15 percent reported two or more other caregivers. Of 249 respondents, 77 percent reported no friends or neighbors in the caring network, and 23 percent reported one or more friends involved.

Attendees ($n = 238$) were asked to indicate their role as caregiver; 56 percent defined themselves as caregivers, and 29 percent reported they were anticipating the caring role. Attendees indicated that the older relatives for whom they were providing care were as follows: 76 percent parents, 8 percent parents-in-law, 4 percent spouses, and 11 percent other relatives, including grandparents, siblings, and aunts.

Caregivers using group services tended to be primarily white, middle-aged, middle-income women of diverse religions and ethnicity. They were primary caregivers for widowed parents over 70 years of age with mild multiple disabilities. There was a disproportionate representation of attendees who were single, given the predominance of married households in the four target areas. As evidenced by the data, they were primarily sole providers of care for their older relatives, and it appears that they lacked informal supports for their own caregiving roles. Therefore they may have been more likely to need peer support and mutual aid from a group.

The Natural Supports Program findings reveal the following:

1. *Organizational Approaches*—The integration of family and aging service networks was beneficial in relation to the diversity of needs of both caregivers and their aging relatives. Program development seems most effective in communities in which both caregivers and their older relatives are living. The NSP not only provided counseling and information to the caregiver, but also was able to mobilize the formal system to provide a variety of services to the older relative, thus supplementing the caregivers' efforts. In cases where caregivers and aged relative live in different communities, program development is facilitated by providing services to caregivers in the community in which the older relative resides.

2. *Programming Considerations*—Factors relating to group composition in terms of the older person(s) of concern were physical, emotional, or mental deterioration; institutional or community-based residence; or residence in caregiver's home, nearby or far away. Factors related to caregivers included their relationship to older person—relative, friend, neighbor; extent of caregiving; demographic characteristics; differential age groupings; size of caring network. Assessments should be made of the training needs of both professional and indigenous group leaders in relation to leadership skills required. Because of the diversity within caregiving situations, it is necessary to identify a specific target group for outreach purposes and program development. An older person's aging process often confronts the caretaker with her or his own aging and mortality. An older relative's need for care can confront the caregiver with longstanding ambivalences regarding the relationship. The need for a service center that could be available to assist caregivers is indicated. The fluctuating nature of caregivers' needs suggest a flexible and comprehensive service approach can meet educational, informational, and supportive needs, as well as provide for short-term task-centered casework intervention.

As to use and value of the groups, both caregivers and professionals expressed the positive value of the group experiences. Some caregivers primarily sought information regarding resources (that proved helpful in finding and using services). Others gained a more realistic understanding of the aging process, enabling them to plan and cope with changes in the caregiving situation. Such understanding helped to assuage fears regarding anticipated physical and mental decline and potential increases in caregiving demands.

Greater toleration and decreased frustration, especially in relation to caring for the mentally impaired, was reported. Caregivers were able to begin addressing their feelings regarding their own aging. Members learned the importance of mutual communication of needs with their older relatives. They developed communications skills that assisted them in involving others in caregiving responsibilities as well as decision-making.

A high degree of interaction and group cohesion developed as a result of caregivers' participation in ongoing small discussion groups. Attendees reported the group programs as the first nonjudgmental, supportive environment in which they could express feelings of anger, frustration, and resentment regarding caregiving roles and responsibilities. Members provided each other with recognition and support for their caring roles. Caregivers were eventually able to recognize and define their limits in caregiving, able to adjust better to new and changing responsibilities as well as to develop coping strategies. Some evidenced skill and knowledge in the area of community resources and entitlements and in functioning as indigenous resource persons. Group sharing for some served as sanctioned opportunity for socialization as well as respite from the caring role.

As Parents Grow Older:
An Intervention Model Program
to Assist Family Caretakers of Elderly Members

The As Parents Grow Older (APGO) program model was implemented and evaluated in several Michigan community sites in an Administration on Aging (AoA) funded project entitled, *The Development and Evaluation of Community Based Support Groups for Families of Aged Persons.*[35] The prototype in the Child and Family Service, Washtenaw County Branch, Child and Family Services of Michigan, Inc. in 1974 developed from a recognition by social workers that adult children caring for aging parents had special needs. These needs, and those of their aging parents, often resulted in tensions and stress for the caretakers.[36, 42]

In order to test the applicability of this program with various caretakers and families living in different communities as well as to develop a training strategy for agency personnel who would serve as program facilitators, a proposal was written by the Institute of Gerontology, The University of Michigan, in collaboration with Child and Family Services of Michigan, Inc. (CFS). Objectives of the 2½-year Model Project included the development and evaluation of a facilitator's manual. In addition, the Project sought "to assess the ability of an existing community structure (Child and Family Services of Michigan, Inc.) to improve services to families with older members through staff development and training."[35]

Purpose and Objectives   The project model, a series of six group sessions, is designed both to help induce supportive behavior in adult children and to provide a link between the parents and community service resources. It is a blend of two traditional interventions and theories—education and learning theory, and counseling and problem-solving models.

The content of the sessions cover sequentially (1) the psychologic aspects of aging, (2) chronic illness and behavioral changes with age, (3) sensory deprivation and communication, (4) alternative living situations and shared decision-making, (5) the availability and utilization of community resources, and (6) dealing with situations and feelings.

The six sessions are designed to provide both practical information to the participants as well as to bring about changes in awareness and understanding of the aging process.

The overall objectives of APGO are to help participants

1. Increase their understanding and knowledge of the aging process;
2. Better understand the emotional reactions and needs of older people;
3. Develop a greater awareness of their responses to their aged relatives and thus their own aging process;
4. Learn to deal more effectively with their own as well as their aged relatives' needs through group problem solving, thus facilitating the development of support systems within the group;
5. Acquire greater access to community supports;
6. Be better able to express and explore alternatives to assist themselves and their aged relatives in maintaining an active and productive way of life.

The prevention and education functions of the APGO model support the premise that despite inherent difficulties families are and will continue to be responsible for supporting their aged members.

Project data support the fact that educational and supportive services are needed to supplement family assistance and strengthen its capacity to care for its elderly members.

The information and concepts provided to the adult child caretakers form a nucleus of educational content of value to physical therapists as well. As noted earlier, medical health service providers will be carrying out their professional duties on behalf of older clients more and more in conjunction with families.

Program Results   Of the family caretakers, 85 percent were female. Men came almost exclusively for their own parents, while women came with concerns about their own as well as their spouses' parents (confirming other findings that the middle-aged woman responds typically to kinship needs). More than 80 percent were facing multiple demands, including outside employment and child care duties, besides devoting a good deal of time to caring for their aging relatives.

The demands faced by these families not only included dual employment, child care, and chores for one aging relative, but in many cases involved care for more than one elder at the same time; 63 percent of respondents reported being concerned about two or more older persons.

The older persons about whom the middle-aged adults were concerned showed various levels of needs. Their ages ranged between 51 and 97 years. Most, 94 percent, had at least one major chronic illness, and 67 percent had three or more chronic conditions. Also, respondents reported that 93 percent of these older persons recently experienced some form of major change in their living arrangements. A majority of the older relatives were widows and in less than perfect health; still, 75 percent of them continued to live independently despite relatively low incomes. Only 14 percent lived with the respondent or siblings of the respondent. The remaining lived under different forms of institutional care.

Nine distinct problems emerged from the project evaluation. There were difficulties that are situational, such as health or informational needs, or problems relating to personal feelings or interpersonal difficulties. Other problems included relations with family members; emotional/behavioral problems; difficulties in communication; difficulties in finding community resources; difficulties in using community resources; the old person's financial situation; or the older person's health.

Based on the subjective reactions of the participants to the APGO model, the program intervention was clearly successful. A total of 91 percent of the participants felt that they had gained in their understanding of the aging process; 78 percent believed they had improved understanding of their older person's needs and feelings; 71 percent reported that they had achieved a greater insight into their own aging. A total of 78 percent of the participants believed they were better prepared to cope with the current and the potential future needs of the elderly, and 81 percent believed that the group process approach, with its combination of information and interpersonal support, proved to be a helpful forum for meeting their needs.[35] Finally, 79 percent indicated that the information and group problem-solving capabilities of their groups seemed most useful.

Every participant experienced improvement in at least one problem area, and 44 percent experienced improvement across four or more of the nine problem areas. Personal feelings showed nearly a 60 percent improvement rate; living arrangements and health problems showed substantially smaller rates of improvement. It seems clear that problems that are more situational may be less amenable to the APGO type of intervention and that APGO is more able to alleviate problems dealing with interpersonal problems, personal adjustment, and problems in communications. When asked how they learned about community programs, 51 percent responded by indicating that it was a direct result of the APGO program.

Perhaps equally relevant for persons working in the medical-health care field was the result of the changes due to improved understanding of the aging process. The project staff developed a true–false test with matched pre–post schedules. Using this instrument, participants showed a decided increase in acquired knowledge.

IMPLICATIONS FOR TRAINING AND SERVICE IN THE FUTURE

The central issue this chapter addresses is the important functions performed by the family kinship or informal support system in caring for the older person, the changing role of the PT in recognition of the family support network with increasing demands on caregivers, and the relationships of both to the formal health–medical care system.

We have examined the essentials in the family support network as the major buttress for the elderly against the losses imposed physiologically and psychologically; this network also serves as the mediating link with sociocultural institutions and systems. A rationale for examining the role of family supports is that it will be increasingly important for the professional provider of health care-medical treatment services to be knowledgeable about family relationships and the elderly. (NOTE: The Joint Commission for The Accreditation of Hospitals mandates evidence of family education as a part of a comprehensive rehabilitation program.)

Although there is no evidence that the value of family care is being adversely affected by postindustrial influences on the family, certain conditions have serious implications for the future. As noted, the increasing numbers of very old persons will affect the family support system. More and more caregivers of elderly family members will themselves be retired or will already experience chronic illness and other losses. There will be the need for new policies dealing with strengthening generational support roles and home care services. More professional training, including that of PTs and others on the rehabilitation team, will be required so that the natural support system can continue in harmony with the formalized system of medical services.

Up until now services for the elderly have been designed primarily for the individual, rather than to include the family network. It has been shown that the family is the chief intermediary between the older person's need for supportive health–medical services and the organized bureaucratic machinery. In fact, past and current policy tends not only to ignore but to undermine the important family support system in helping elderly persons remain self-sufficient. More attention will be directed in the future toward finding ways to encourage a workable, harmonious balance between the family network system and the formal service systems.

Sociocultural changes also are affecting the critically important role of family caregiver for the elderly parents and relatives. One concern for future support is that the female caregiver is more and more engaged in work–career roles. It has been shown that problems of stress for the caregivers are exacerbated by responsibilities of work in addition to those of the family. Factors that might offset this trend are complex but include the changing role of husband or father in the household, in sharing child caregiving tasks, and in household tasks. Could this affect the future role of son/son-in-law in the caregiving function so that he would assume more filial responsibility for personal care and emotional support?

It has been shown that educational support programs benefit the caregivers in helping them to understand aging changes for parents, to understand their own aging process, and to learn how to utilize the community support services to better advantage for the elderly. Educational programs in the future could be directed to husbands and sons or could involve both spouses in a team approach. Similarly, the education system preparing future professionals will be more cognizant of trends in family support and of research studies probing emerging developments in age-related medical and health care services.

It has been suggested that a high level of professional training will be required also for the PT to be aware of the elderly person's needs to maintain individual status within the family as well as make decisions and have a positive attitude toward improvement and the ability to take advantage of community support systems. Reciprocity in the family relationships may extend to the PT in the future, when rehabilitation involves more and more services within the family network system. Increasing involvement will include roles advising family members and assisting adult children in caring for physically dependent elderly in a home setting. Education needs for the PT in working with elderly patients and family members, as noted, include understanding one's own aging as well as the aging process itself; understanding the roles of family caretakers; realizing the need to make a controlled investment in the elderly patient; and developing a cooperative relationship with the patient's family members.

Investigation into the relationship of the professional and the family support system as it emerges on behalf of elderly patients will be especially valuable. Future research data will in turn be of value to training institutions, so that curricula may be revised to incorporate these data into the important aspects of professional practice. It is anticipated that professional organizations also will recognize the relevancy of training in geriatrics and assist schools and colleges to establish opportunities for certification or continuing professional education programs for practicing physical therapists.

REFERENCES

1. Silverstone B: An overview of research on informal supports: implications for policy and practice. Gerontological Society Meeting, Dallas, 1978.
2. Litwak E: Extended Kin relations in an industrial democratic society. In: Social Structure and the Family: Generational Relations, eds. Shanas E, Streib G. Prentice-Hall, Englewood-Cliffs, N.J., 1965.
3. Sussman MB: The family life of old people. In: Handbook of Aging and the Social Sciences, eds. Binstock R, Shanas E. Van Nostrand Reinhold, New York, 1976.
4. Tabak HL: The role of the family. J Am Health Care Assoc 1979.
5. Lebowitz BD: Old age and family functioning. J Gerontol Social Work, 1(2):111–118, 1978.
6. Califano JA Jr: The aging of America: Questions for the four-generation society. Annals AAPSS 438:96–107, Jul 1978.
7. Blenkner M: Social work and family relationships in later life with some thoughts on filial maturity. In: Social Structure and the Family: Generational Relations, eds. Shanas E, Streib G. Prentice-Hall, Englewood-Cliffs, N.J., 1965, pp. 46–59.
8. Lewis MA, Binstock R, Cantor M, Schneewind E: The extent to which informal and formal supports interact to maintain the older people in the community. Gerontological Society Annual Meeting, San Diego, 1980.
9. Hawker M: Geriatrics for Physiotherapists and the Allied Professions. Queen Square, London, 1974.
10. McClusky HY: Education for aging: the scope of the field and perspectives for the future. In: Education for the Aging, eds. Grabowski SM, Mason D. ERIC Clearinghouse on Adult Education, Syracuse, N.Y., 1974.
11. Tibbitts C: Middle-aged and older people in American society. In: Planning Welfare Services for Older People. Dept. HEW, Washington, D.C., 1965.
12. Hilliboe HE: A modern pattern for meeting the health needs of the aging. In: The New Frontiers of Aging, eds. Donahue W, Tibbitts C. The University of Michigan Press, Ann Arbor, 1957, pp. 45–62.
13. Tibbitts C: Can we invalidate negative stereotypes of aging? Gerontologist 19(1), 1979.

14. Thompson WE, Streib G: Meaningful activity in a family context. In: Aging and Leisure: A Research Perspective into the Meaningful Use of Time, ed. Kleemeier RW. Oxford University Press, New York, 1961.
15. Troll LE: The family of later life: A decade review. Marriage Family J May 1971.
16. Cantor MH: Neighbors and friends; An overlooked resource in the informal support system. Gerontological Society Meeting, San Francisco, 1977.
17. Shanas E, Streib G: Social structure and the family: Generational relations, ed. Shanas E, Streib G. Prentice-Hall, Englewood Cliffs, N.H., 1965.
18. Shanas E: Social myth as hypothesis; The case of the family relations of old people. Gerontologist 19(1), 1979.
19. Blenkner M: The normal dependencies of aging. In: The Dependencies of Old People, ed. Kalish R. Institute of Gerontology, Ann Arbor, 1969, pp. 27–37.
20. Kreps J: The economics of intergenerational relationships. In: Social Structure and the Family: Generational Relations, eds. Shanas E, Streib G. Prentice-Hall, New York, 1965.
21. Donahue W: Psychological changes with advancing age. In: Planning Welfare Services for Older People, Washington, D.C., 1965.
22. Clark M: Is dependency in old age culture bound? Gerontological Society Meeting, 1967.
23. Sicker M: Some thoughts on a national policy for long-term care. Gerontological Social Work J 2(3):271–275, 1980.
24. Shanas E: The unmarried old person in the United States: Living arrangements and care in illness, myth, and fact. International Social Science Research Seminar in Gerontology, Sweden, 1963.
25. Sussman MB, Burchinal L: Kin family network: Unheralded structure in current conceptualizations of family functioning. Marriage Family Living 24:231–240, 1962.
26. Blazer D: Working with the elderly patient's family. Geriatrics 33:117–123, 1978.
27. Comptroller General of United States: The well-being of older people in Cleveland, Ohio. U.S. General Accounting Office, April 19, 1977.
28. US Dept of Health, Education, and Welfare, National Center for Health Statistics. Home Health Care for Persons 55 Years and Over. Vital and Health Statistics Publication Series 10, no. 73, 1972.
29. Population Reference Bureau, Inc., 1975.
30. Adams BN: Interaction theory and the social network. Sociometry 30:64–78, 1967.
31. Shanas E: A note on restriction of life space: Attitudes of age cohorts. Hlth Social Behav J 9:86–90, 1968.
32. Schmidt MG: Failing parents, aging children. Gerontol Social Work J 2(3):259–268, 1980.
33. Brody EM, Spark GM: Institutionalization of the aged: A family crisis. Family Process 5(1):76–90, 1966.
34. Hess B, Waring J: Parent and child in later life: Rethinking the relationship. In: Child Influences on Marital and Family Interactions: A Lifespan Perspective, eds. Lernez R, Spanier B. Academic Press, New York, 1978, 241–273.
35. Brahce CI, Silverman AG, Leon J: Altering a service delivery system to improve family care of the elderly: final report. Ann Arbor: Institute of Gerontology, 1981.
36. Silverman AG, Brahce CI: "As Parents Grow Older": An Intervention Model. Gerontol Social Work J 2(1):77–85, 1979.
37. The aged and community mental health: A guide to program development. Formulated by the Committee on Aging. Group for the Advancement of Psychiatry, Vol 8. New York, 1971.

38. Milloy M: Casework with the older person and his family. Social Casework J pp 450–455, Oct 1964.
39. Campbell R, Chenoweth B, Kraus C: Peer supports for older adults, manual for replication. Turner Geriatric Clinic, University of Michigan Hospital, Ann Arbor, 1981.
40. Crossman L, London C, Barry C: Older women caring for disabled spouses: A model for supportive services. Gerontologist 21(5):464–470, 1981.
41. Hudis IE, Guchsbaum MD: Components of community based group programs for strengthening family supports to their aging relatives: implications for replication. Community Service Society of New York, Gerontological Society Meeting, Dallas, 1978.
42. Kahn BH, Silverman AG: Family service highlights. Family Serv Assoc Am 2(5), 1976.

8 | Cardiac Considerations and Physical Training

Louis R. Amundsen   *Marian L. Eliason*
Corinne T. Ellingham *Louvain G. Arndts*

Prior to embarking on a physical therapy program for an elderly patient, it is necessary to determine that the patient needs exercise, that the cardiovascular effort is likely to be safe and beneficial, and that the subject is motivated and interested in physical training. In order to utilize effective and safe exercise intensity levels it is necessary to evaluate the capacity for exercise of each individual who will participate in a physical therapy program. This is especially crucial with the elderly patient population because they have an increased susceptibility to the secondary complication of bed-rest deconditioning. In order for the physical therapy and rehabilitation program to be administered safely, it is necessary to determine the safe limits of exercise for every elderly patient. The assessment of exercise capacity must be sensitive enough to detect small changes and must be specific to the goals of the treatment program.

Cardiovascular evaluation and training methods should be convenient, inexpensive, and progressive in difficulty and intensity. These methods should also be easily adapted to the needs of the well, the frail, and the disabled elderly. There is also a need to be reasonably certain that a proposed training regimen will be effective.

The literature review and pilot study described in this chapter provide an overview of cardiopulmonary evaluation and training for elderly up to the age of 75 and extrapolate implications for evaluation and training approached for the very old (over 80 years of age).

NEED FOR EXERCISE FOR THE ELDERLY

Elderly individuals need cardiovascular endurance training and instruction concerning appropriate activity levels because they tend to be inactive and to have an increased incidence of conditions that require supervised training, e.g., heart and respiratory disease, obesity, chronic pain, arthritis, peripheral vascular problems, cerebrovascular accidents, diabetes.[1-4]

Activity levels of the "healthy" elderly have been estimated. The energy expenditures of older workers is the same as that of younger workers during the working day; however, a study of the male population of Tecumseh, Michigan indicated that the frequency of participation in leisure activities decreased rapidly after age 40. Time spent swimming, bowling, fishing, dancing, and hunting decreased rapidly with increasing age. Walking and lawn-mowing with a power mower decreased after age 60. Gardening increased with age in the study sample (up to age 65).[4]

Sidney and Shephard[5] reported that a group of elderly university employees rarely reached or exceeded a heart rate of 120 beats per minute (bpm). A heart rate of 120 bpm is likely to represent the training intensity threshold for older employed individuals. Other studies of representative groups of men and women over the age of 65 indicate that the drastic reduction of physical activity observed in middle-aged men continues in the population over age 65.

For the frail and/or disabled elderly the ill effects of bed rest are well documented. Deficiencies in endurance and strength are a common consequence of prolonged bed rest, reduced mobility, and cardiopulmonary disease. Bed rest and inactivity will produce detrimental effects even when no other pathologic process is involved. Bed rest results in decreases in muscle strength, bone density, blood volume, and orthostatic tolerance.[6-8] Aerobic power will decrease dramatically after 3 weeks of bed rest for normal young healthy subjects.[6] Even 10 to 11 days of chair rest by healthy subjects causes decreases in work capacity and orthostatic tolerance.[9] It is obvious that activity levels tend to decrease with advancing age and that inactivity will promote physiologic deterioration.

FEASIBILITY OF TRAINING

If the premise is accepted that an optimal level of physical activity will minimize or eliminate the detrimental effects of inactivity in young normal subjects and in cardiac patients,[10-13] then we still need to know if increasing the physical activity levels of the elderly will be beneficial. The specific effects of aging on skeletal muscle, on the cardiopulmonary system, and on the decline in bone mass have been reviewed[14-18] (see also Chapter 2). All of these changes are similar to the physiologic deterioration caused by inactivity. However, aging per se does cause deterioration independent of the effects of inactivity. Even though the effects of aging will increase the risk and decrease the effectiveness of training, the feasibility of effective cardiopulmonary training for the elderly has been demonstrated.[19-23]

Logically, the key to effective training is the utilization of appropriate exercise intensity levels. These exercise intensities must be based on the exercise capacity of the individual being trained, on the use of exercises that are appropriate for these individuals, and on the functional analysis of the activity of the individual patient. A training program requires a pretraining evaluation, the use of exercises with known intensity levels, patient education to translate effort into implications for activities of daily living, and frequent assessment during training sessions.

ASSESSING EXERCISE CAPACITY

When assessing exercise capacity it is necessary to know the normal and abnormal cardiovascular responses to physical exercise.[24,25] In the young the cardiovascular and pulmonary systems respond quickly to acute exercise by increasing heart rate, respiratory rate, stroke volume, tidal volume, and blood flow to active tissue. Advanced aging or progressive disease will lengthen the time required to reach steady state or homeostasis during exercise at a given intensity level.[26]

An equilibrium or steady-state condition will be reached if the functional reserve capacities of the cardiovascular and pulmonary systems have not been exceeded, however.[27] The exercise load that requires more oxygen and energy substrate, glucose, and free fatty acids than the cardiopulmonary systems are able to deliver can be identified when work loads are gradually increased. It is of course necessary to recognize the signs and symptoms of exercise intolerance early enough to prevent undue discomfort or risk to the patient. Prior to initiation of the exercise evaluation, the patient should demonstrate the ability to meet the demands of the resting state. The resting pulse rate should be between 60 and 100 bpm. If the heart rate is faster or slower than this range or is irregular, the resting electrocardiogram will need to be interpreted. Any unstable rhythm, ventricular arrhythmias, or ST segment shifts would contraindicate exercise testing or training.[24,25] Ideally, even for elderly subjects the resting systolic blood pressure should be between 100 and 150 mmHg.[28] However, pressures greater than 150 mmHg are common for the elderly and do not necessarily prevent safe exercise. If the resting pressure exceeds 225 mmHg, however, exercise evaluation should not be started. At resting pressures approaching 225 mmHg greater caution and lower and smaller exercise levels and increments should be used.

A detailed description of the physical assessment and what to look for in a medical history concerning cardiovascular phenomena have been described previously in this series.[29]

The heart rate normally increases as the work rate increases, but in the elderly the rate of increase will be greater and/or the maximal heart rate observed will be lower (see Figure 8-1 and Figure 8-2).[30-32] Normal active individuals at any age will have a slower increase in heart rate than sedentary subjects or cardiac

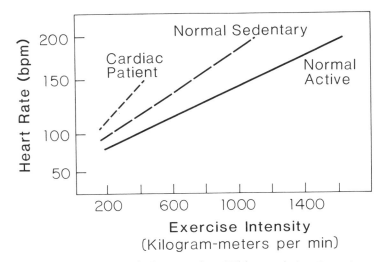

Fig. 8-1. Heart rate responses during exercise. (With permission from Amundsen LR (ed): Cardiac Rehabilitation. Churchill Livingstone, New York, 1981.)

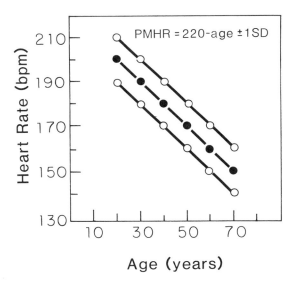

Fig. 8-2. Predicted maximal heart rate (PMHR). (With permission from Amundsen LR (ed): Cardiac Rehabilitation. Churchill Livingstone, New York, 1981.)

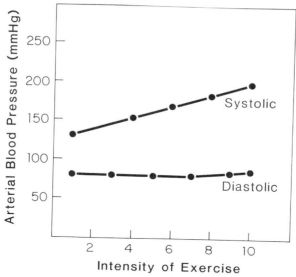

Fig. 8-3. Typical blood pressure response to progressively increasing work rates, METs (metabolic equivalents: 3.5 ml O_2/min/kg). (With permission from Amundsen LR (ed): Cardiac Rehabilitation. Churchill Livingstone, New York, 1981.)

patients.[30] Even at equivalent ages cardiac patients will usually have lower maximal heart rates than individuals with normal hearts. The maximal heart rate decreases as a function of age (see Figure 8-2).[30-32] The predicted maximal heart rate (PMHR) plus or minus one standard deviation is equal to 220 minus the age in years.[33]

Blood pressure responses also can and should be used to assess responses to exercise (see Figure 8-3). Rhythmic isotonic exercise of the lower extremities should cause large increases in systolic blood pressure but only minimal changes in diastolic pressure (Figure 8-3).[34] An increase of 7.5 mmHg per metabolic equivalent (MET) is considered normal for systolic pressure. If the systolic blood pressure (SBP) increases more than 12 mmHg or less than 5 mmHg per MET, the response is considered hypertensive or hypotensive, respectively.[35]

If the SBP fails to increase or falls when the exercise intensity is increased, the heart as a pump and/or the cardiovascular system as a shunt is failing, which of course requires stopping or decreasing the intensity of the exercise. In order to minimize chances of overworking the heart or risking arterial rupture or aneurysm formation, the SBP should not exceed 225 mmHg;[36] however, values up to 300 mmHg have been observed during exercise without apparent untoward effects.[37]

In the young normal individual the diastolic blood pressure (DBP) should change very little as the intensity of ambulation, bicycling, or treadmill walking increases.[34] Elderly subjects, even those classified as well elderly, are very likely to demonstrate increases in DBP in response to exercise. If the DBP exceeds 130 mmHg exercise should be stopped or the intensity should be decreased.[24,38] Decreasing the intensity of exercise is preferable to completely stopping it because continuing activity will promote the continued contribution of the auxiliary peripheral blood pumps, especially the gastrocnemius-soleus muscle group, and the respiratory system's contribution to venous return. If it is necessary to stop exercise completely, the elderly individual should sit or lie in a head-up or Fowler's position. This position will prevent sudden overfilling of the heart and minimize the risk of promoting further heart failure due to excessive preload.

During physical exercise the therapist should estimate the adequacy of regional blood flow by observing skin color, changes in coordination, and levels of alertness. The cheeks, earlobes, and nose should become pinker as the duration and intensity of exercise increases.[24] If these areas suddenly turn pale, the exercise intensity should be decreased. One can be relatively certain that the blood flow to the kidney and liver is being sacrificed in an attempt to maintain blood flow to the working muscles, the heart, and the brain when sudden pallor is accompanied by falling systolic blood pressure.

Pain and discomfort, such as angina pectoris, dyspnea, intermittent claudication, or joint pain, are also likely to be observed in the elderly and are reasons for decreasing/stopping a bout of exercise[24] or finding other evaluation procedures that do not cause lower extremity pain (e.g., upper extremity ergometry).

After exercise the heart rate, blood pressure, and respiration should return rapidly to near-resting levels. The heart rate is expected to return to approximately 100 bpm within 6 minutes after exercise ceases.[39] Blood pressure, cognition, equilibrium, and skin color should be observed during the first 5 minutes of recovery after exercise in order to detect excessive pooling of blood in the lower extremities.[36]

These principles need to be applied in assessing tolerance for any exercise, especially when functional capacity is being determined prior to initiating an exercise training program for elderly subjects.

Working capacity is usually expressed as maximal aerobic power and determined by submaximal or by symptom-limited progressive exercise tolerance testing.[40–42] It is possible to determine maximal aerobic power in elderly subjects by conducting tests with the classical criteria developed on young normal subjects for

Table 8-1. Submaximal Exercise Test Protocol for Elderly Subjects

Exercise Stage	Duration (min)	Total Time (min)	METs[a]
1	3	3	2
2	3	6	3
3	3	9	4
4[b]	3	12	5
5	3	15	6
6	3	18	7

[a] Metabolic equivalents.
[b] Rarely achieved by subjects over age 75.

Table 8-2. Metabolic Equivalents (METs) of Bicycle Ergometer Work Loads

Work Load		MET According to Body Weight (kg)							
Watts	kpm/min[a]	50	60	70	80	90	100	110	120
10	60	2.1	2.0	1.9	1.9	1.8	1.8	1.8	1.8
25	150	3.0	2.8	2.6	2.5	2.4	2.3	2.2	2.1
50	300	4.6	4.1	3.7	3.4	3.2	3.0	2.9	2.8
75	450	6.1	5.4	4.8	4.4	4.1	3.8	3.6	3.4
100	600	7.7	6.6	5.9	5.4	4.9	4.6	4.3	4.1
125	750	9.2	7.9	7.0	6.3	5.8	5.4	5.0	4.7
150	900	10.8	9.2	8.1	7.3	6.6	6.1	5.7	5.4
175	1050	12.3	10.5	9.2	8.3	7.5	6.9	6.4	6.0
200	1200	13.8	11.8	10.3	9.2	8.4	7.7	7.1	6.6
250	1500	16.9	14.4	12.5	11.1	10.1	9.2	8.5	7.9
300	1800	20.0	16.9	14.7	13.1	11.8	10.8	9.9	9.2

The test protocol is given in Table 8-1.
[a] Kilopond meters per minute are equivalent to kilogram meters per minute.

the establishment of maximal aerobic power.[43] Since progressive increase of work loads until an increase in work rate no longer causes an increase in oxygen uptake is perceived as extremely stressful and sometimes is impossible to achieve in young normal sedentary adults, this procedure is not reasonable for elderly individuals, who are more likely to be sedentary and to possess hidden cardiovascular disorders. In our opinion the test used must be safe and intense enough to allow an accurate estimate of maximal aerobic power and tolerance for the intensity levels to be used for physical therapy training.

We have used the exercise protocol given in Table 8-1 for evaluating well and frail elderly individuals. Table 8-2 provides the conversions between metabolic equivalents and bicycle ergometer work loads.[38,41] Table 8-3 lists the metabolic equivalents for treadmill walking.[35] Tables 8-4 and 8-5 contain MET values for the step ergometer and for walking on a firm surface.[35,41,44] Any of these modes of exercise can and have been used for testing the elderly[17,26,43] with functional lower extremity function. While many functional evaluations have been used to assess activities of daily living and related functional ability, only one test was located based on physiologic phenomena.[45–52] The Kottke-Kubicek Five Stage Activity Test can be used to quantify physiologic responses to functional activities.[52] Our adaptation of this test is illustrated in Figures 8-4 and 8-5 and is described in detail later in this chapter.

Table 8-3. Submaximal Treadmill Exercise Test

Exercise Stage	Duration (min)	Total Time (min)	Treadmill Speed (mph)	Percent Grade (% incline)	METs
1	3	3	2.0	0.0	2
2	3	6	2.0	3.5	3
3	3	9	2.0	7.0	4
4[a]	3	12	2.0	10.5	5
5	3	15	2.0	14.0	6
6	3	18	2.0	17.5	7

[a] Rarely achieved by the elderly.

Table 8-4. Submaximal Progressive Step Test, 24 Ascents per Minute

Exercise Stage	Duration (min)	Total Time (min)	Step Height (cm)	METs
1	3	3	0	2.2
2	3	6	5	3.0
3	3	9	12	4.0
4	3	12	18	5.0
5	3	15	25	6.0
6	3	18	32	7.0

TRAINING METHODS

Most studies of the effectiveness of training the elderly have demonstrated that subjects with an average age of 65 years can be trained by jogging and by riding bicycle ergometers.[53–58] Subjects of these studies and most individuals 65 to 75 years of age are functioning independently in the community. Individuals 75 to 85 years old often require some support or assistance from family members or community resources. Individuals 85 years of age or older usually need considerable assistance and are most likely to require professional supportive services (nursing-home care or home care).[57] Obviously arbitrary divisions based on chronologic age alone are not appropriate; however, these chronologic and functional divisions can be used to classify existing literature and to plan exercise testing and training regimens for elderly people.

Very little information is available that evaluates the effectiveness or safety of given exercise levels for subjects over the age of 75.[57,58] However, it is likely that individuals over the age of 75 and the frail elderly will benefit from training levels based on principles developed from research on normal young subjects, cardiac patients, the well elderly, and the young old.[11–13,33,59–61] It has been demonstrated that exercise intensities of 60 to 75 percent of maximal aerobic power will be sufficient to produce training effects in previously untrained subjects in these categories. Given that individuals 65 to 75 years old can be expected to have maximal aerobic power of 5 to 7 METs and that ambulatory nursing home populations have demonstrated maximums of 2 to 4 METs,[61] it is possible to select and predict activities that will be effective for training subjects older than 75 years. Walking, stationary bicycling, stationary stepping, light calisthenics, and various recreational activities, and activities of daily living (ADL) are likely to be appropriate, see Tables 8-6 and 8-7.[61–69] Calisthenic exercises of known low-intensity levels

Table 8-5. Submaximal Walking Test

Exercise Stage	Duration (min)	Total Time (min)	Speed MPH	m/min^{-1}	METs
1	3	3	1.5	40.2	2.2
2	3	6	2.5	67.1	3.0
3	3	9	3.0	80.5	3.5
4	3	12	3.5	93.9	4.1
5[a]	3	15	4.0	107.3	4.8

[a] Rarely achieved by the elderly.

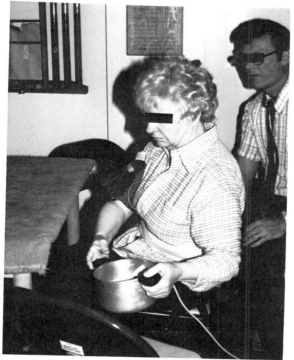

Fig. 8-4.   Simulated kitchen task.

have been described previously in this series[41,68] and are discussed along with a model program later in this chapter. MET levels have been determined for calisthenics by others,[63-66] but these values are meaningful only when determined at steady state or when the methods of the original literature report are duplicated. METs measured at steady state can be used for any time interval, usually 1 to 3 minutes per exercise, but MET values determined over short durations—e.g., 30 seconds or 1 minute—can be applied only to exercise of the same duration.

When training heart rates are determined by the method first described by Karvonen,[11,70] the percentage of maximal heart rate will usually be acheived when exercising at the same percentage of maximal aerobic power. This is not true when the percentage of maximal heart rate is based on a starting point of zero. When a zero base is used, higher percentages of maximal heart rate are required to reach 60 to 75 percent of maximal aerobic power.[36]

PILOT STUDY

The goal was to identify practical exercise regimens effective for increasing the capacity of the elderly to perform activities of daily living. Effective training should decrease the physiologic effort required to perform any activity the subject is now

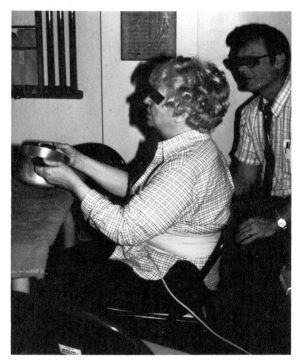

Fig. 8-5.   Monitoring physiologic responses during the simulated kitchen task.

able to complete, increase the number of activities the subject is able to perform, and delay the onset of dependent living. The immediate objective of this pilot study was to test and compare the effectiveness of the following exercise regimens: (1) aerobic calisthenics and (2) walking/stair climbing.

These exercise regimens were chosen because they provide very convenient and inexpensive exercise training methods that require little or no equipment and are especially applicable to group exercise. Calisthenics have the added advantage of requiring a minimum of space and of training all major muscle groups of the body. Since training is expected to decrease the cardiac effort of performing the specific movement being trained, a set of calisthenics that involves the movement of most parts of the body is likely to decrease the cardiac effort of a wide variety of activities needed for activities of daily living.

The effectiveness of these two trained regimens for increasing aerobic power and decreasing cardiac effort during a simulated kitchen task was tested and compared. The effects of training on body weight, spontaneous physical activity, and on selected psychologic phenomena were also tested.

Twenty-three female residents of a high-rise apartment administered by the Minneapolis Housing Authority volunteered for the study. The Minneapolis Housing Authority administers 43 high-rise apartment complexes with approximately 6000 residents. Disabled persons or people over the age of 62 are eligible.

Table 8-6. Approximate Energy Requirements of Physical Activities

Activity	METs
Self-care activities and physical exercises in bed with back supported	
Feeding self	1–1.5
Washing hands and face	1–1.5
Washing body while sitting in a chair (excluding back and legs)	1.7
Brushing teeth	1–1.5
Care of fingernails	1–1.5
Shaving	1.6
Combing hair	1.6
Passive ROM[a] exercises to all extremities	1.0
Active ROM[a] exercises to all extremities	1.0–1.5
Active ROM[a] exercises with moderate resistance to all extremities	1.5–2.0
Calisthenics (by author)	
Weise	2.2–10.3
Fletcher	1.4–4.2
Kellerman	2.2–6.9
Greer	2.0–4.5
Amundsen	1.7–5.9

Includes resting metabolic needs.
[a] ROM, range of motion.

The average age is 76.5 years (range 53 to 92); 8 percent of this population is under age 62 and disabled. The sample of 23 had an average age of 70.7 (range 57 to 80). All subjects signed an informed consent statement and completed a medical history form, which was reviewed by a physician. The subjects were medically stable but did not appear to be unusually healthy. The following medical conditions were present in one to eight subjects at the start of the study: blindness, rheumatoid arthritis, stable angina, peripheral vascular disorders, emphysema, asthma, orthopedic conditions, and hypertension.

All subjects were invited to attend a preliminary session designed to provide for practice pedaling of a bicycle ergometer. One week later during a single evaluation session subjects were weighed and measured, completed questionnaires concerning physical activity and state anxiety, and performed a bicycle ergometer test and the modified Kottke-Kubicek Five Stage Activity Test. A physical activity questionnaire was adapted from the form used by Cassel.[71] Anxiety levels were measured with the State and Trait Anxiety Inventory form STAI-1.[72]

The bicycle test protocol is given in Tables 8-1 and 8-2. This test consisted of a series of 3 minute exercise bouts. The first bout or level was always performed at a 2-MET intensity. Exercise intensity was increased in 1-MET increments until the subject asked to stop, some sign of exercise intolerance occurred, or the HR exceeded 75 percent of the available HR range. This 75 percent level approximates the 85 percent level when a zero-based percentage of maximal heart rate is used.

The Kottke-Kubicek Activity Test (simulated kitchen task) was modified to consist only of moving a weighted kettle from a 30-inch high table to a chair on the right of the subject, returning it to the table, moving it to a chair on the left of the subject, and returning it to the table (see Figures 8-4 and 8-5). This test was

Table 8-7. Approximate Energy Requirements of Physical Activities

Category	Self-Care or Home	Occupational	Recreational[b]	Physical Conditioning
Very light (<3 METs)	Washing, shaving, dressing Desk work, writing Washing dishes Driving auto	Sitting (clerical, assembling) Standing (store clerk, bartender) Driving truck[a] Crane operator[a]	Shuffleboard Horseshoes Bait casting Billiards Archery Golf (cart)	Walking (level at 2 mph) Stationary bicycle (very low resistance) Very light calisthenics
Light 3–5 METs	Cleaning windows Raking leaves Weeding Power lawn mowing Waxing floors (slowly) Painting Carrying objects (15–30 lb)	Stocking shelves (light objects) Light welding Light carpentry[b] Machine assembly Auto repair Paper hanging	Dancing (social and square) Golf (walking) Sailing Horseback riding Volleyball (6 man) Tennis (doubles)	Walking (3–4 mph) Level bicycling (6–8 mph) Light calisthenics
Moderate 5–7 METs	Easy digging in garden Level hand lawn mowing Climbing stairs (slowly) Carrying objects (30–60 lb)	Carpentry (exterior home building)[b] Shoveling dirt[b] Pneumatic tools[b]	Badminton (competitive) Tennis (singles) Snow skiing (downhill) Light backpacking Basketball Football Skating (ice and roller) Horseback riding (gallop)	Walking (4.5–5 mph) Bicycling (9–10 mph) Swimming (breast stroke)

Includes resting metabolic needs.
[a] May cause added psychologic stress that will increase work load on the heart.
[b] May produce disproportionate myocardial demands because of use of arms or isometric exercise. Modified from Haskell WL: Design and implementation of cardiac conditioning programs. In: Rehabilitation of the Coronary Patient, eds. Wenger NK, Hellerstein HK. Wiley, New York, 1978. Reprinted by permission of John Wiley & Sons, Inc.

performed at a rate of 30 moves per minute. Each full cycle, from the table to the chair and back to the table, requires four moves. This test also consisted of a series of 3 minute bouts or levels. Level 1 was always performed with the kettle weighing 3.5 lb (1½ kg). After 1 minute of rest the subject was allowed to progress to 5.5 lb (2½ kg) if no signs or symptoms of exercise intolerance were observed or reported. Subjects progressed to 8.5 lb (4 kg) if the previous exercise levels were performed without exceeding the target heart rate or causing any indices of exercise intolerance.

Heart rate was recorded during the last 10 seconds of the third minute of each exercise level (see Figure 8-6). Blood pressure was recorded immediately after each level of the kettle test and during the last 15 seconds of each level of the bicycle ergometer test.

The subjects who completed the pretraining evaluation were divided into high- and low-intensity groups and randomly assigned to the calisthenics or the walking group. The calisthenics are described in Figure 8-7, and the progression

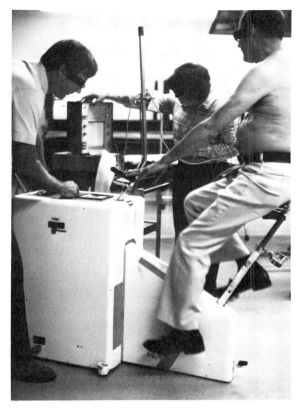

Fig. 8-6.   Progressive exercise tolerance testing: electrocardiogram.

plan is given in Table 8-8. The calisthenics were performed at the following counts per minute (CPM):

Side bends	60
Push-push	120
Pull-pull	120
Alternate-leg raises	120
Toe touch–almost	60
Arm lifts	120
Side bends—one arm	60
Arm swings	120
Stepping	80, 100, and 120

The energy cost of stepping at 80, 100, and 120 CPM is shown in Table 8-9.

The training regimen for walking/stair climbing is outlined in Table 8-10. The high-rise apartment selected for this study contains stairways at two ends of

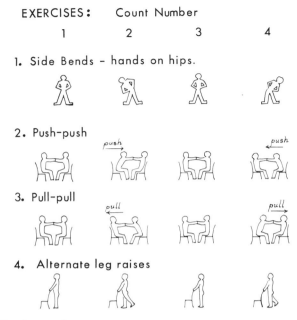

EXERCISES: Count Number

1   2   3   4

1. Side Bends – hands on hips.

2. Push-push

3. Pull-pull

4. Alternate leg raises

Fig. 8-7.   Calisthenic exercises.

the building and balconies around two atria (see Figure 8-8 and 8-9) that provide a pleasant and convenient place to walk.

Target heart rates were set at 60 to 75 percent of the expected heart rate range. For a zero-based range this corresponds to 70 to 85 percent of the predicted maximal heart rate. However, target heart rates were never set higher than heart rates achieved during the bicycle ergometer test. Pulse rates were monitored at rest prior to each training session, during the last one third or immediately after each training session, and after 5 minutes of recovery. Subjects were taught to

Table 8-8. Exercise Program: Calisthenics

Week	Number of Exercises	Duration per Exercise (min)	Total Time (min)
1	1–9, 1	1	10
2	1–9, 1	1	10
3	1–9, 1	2	20
4	1–9, 1	2	20
5	1–9, 1	3	30
6	1–9, 1	3	30
7	1–9, 1	3	30
8	1–9, 1	3	30
9	1–9, 1	3	30
10	1–9, 1	3	30

An 8-oz (0.4-kg) weight (hand held) was added to exercises 6 to 8 for high-capacity subjects (done bilaterally).

Table 8-9. Metabolic Equivalents (METs) of Step Ergometer Work

Height	Stepping Frequency		
(inches)	20/min	25/min	30/min
0	2.0	2.4	2.8
4	3.4	4.0	4.5
8	4.7	5.9	7.0
12	6.1	7.8	9.5

Adapted from references 38 and 41.

monitor their own radial pulse. The subjects were generally able to determine accurate pulse counts at rest but tended to report falsely low exercise counts. We believe that the subjects were able to count accurately, but were slow to locate the pulse after exercise, which would of course result in counts lower than those determined by the therapists.

Exercise sessions were supervised by physical and occupational therapy instructors and graduate students. Supervised sessions were provided on Monday and Thursday for 9 weeks. Subjects were encouraged to exercise one additional session each week.

Results of the Pilot Study

Maximal aerobic power was estimated by extrapolation from the results of the submaximal bicycle ergometer test. This estimate was based on the expected linear increase in heart rate as work load increased and on the predicted maximal heart rate.[41] The average maximal aerobic power of the eight subjects who completed training by the walking/stair climbing method increased from 4.5 to 6.0 METs after 9 weeks of training ($p < 0.01$). The eight subjects who completed the calisthenics regimen increased from a mean of 3.6 to 4.7 METs ($p < 0.05$). The gains of these two groups were not different ($p > 0.05$). Four subjects who did not train showed no significant change in maximal aerobic power (3.7 to 3.8 METs; $p > 0.05$). Physical activity scores increased from a mean of 9.6 to 11.5 ($p < 0.05$).

Table 8-10. Exercise Program: Walking/Stair Climbing

Week	Distance (miles)	Stairs[a] (loops)	Speed (mph)	Total Time (min)
1	0.3	0–2	2	10
2	0.50	0–4	2	14
3	0.70	0–6	2.5	16
4	0.80	0–6	2.5	20
5	1.00	0–8	2.5	25
6	1.20	0–8	2.5	30
7	1.30	0–10	2.6	30
8	1.40	0–10	2.8	30
9	1.50	0–12	3	30
10	1.60	0–12	3.2	30

[a] Each stair loop consisted of one to six flights of stairs followed by level walking.

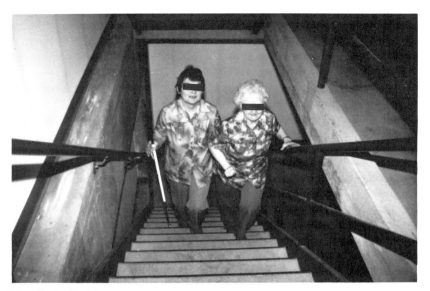

Fig. 8-8.   Stair climbing.

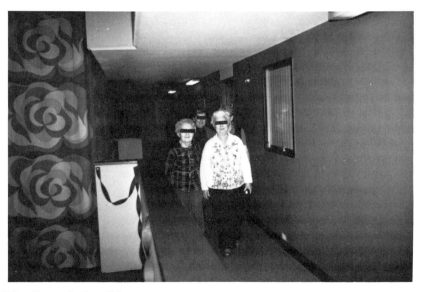

Fig. 8-9.   Supervised walking.

State anxiety scores were generally in the low normal range for the subjects who completed the training program and did not appear to change after training. When only the low-capacity subjects are considered, the calisthenics regimen caused larger decreases in heart rate responses at a given work rate on the simulated kitchen task than did the walking/stair climbing regimen. The calisthenics regimen appears to provide more relevant changes in the cardiopulmonary capacity to perform upper-extremity-dominated ADL.

Pretraining aerobic power was higher than that reported for ambulatory nursing home populations. Posttraining values are comparable with values expected for the young old (5 to 7 METs).

This appears to be the only study that documents the effectiveness of calisthenics for increasing the aerobic capacity of the elderly. Kellerman et al.[66] reported that a training regimen consisting only of calisthenics did not increase the functional capacity of patients with angina pectoris.

Previous work by other investigators has demonstrated that jogging or riding stationary bicycles will improve the functional capacity of subjects with an average age of up to 65 years.[19-23] Reports concerning subjects older than an average of 65 years of age are rare. Smith et al.[73] have trained older female subjects ($\bar{x}$ 83 years of age) using low-intensity calisthenic style activities. In the Smith study bone mineral loss was reversed in the trained group, but changes in functional capacity were not reported.

CONCLUSION

This review of the literature and pilot study description indicate that elderly individuals are usually less than optimally active but are able to improve cardiopulmonary response to exercise through training. Pretraining evaluations capable of safely and specifically determining safe levels of physical therapy were recommended. Training regimens and training intensities appropriate for medically stable elderly individuals were presented; these methods were especially effective for subjects with the following medical conditions: blindness, stable angina, peripheral vascular disorders, emphysema, and hypertension. The training regimens were readily adaptable to subjects with various orthopedic problems and for a subject with rheumatoid arthritis.

With the rapidly increasing population of elderly over the age of 75, and therefore the increasing frequency of lower-extremity dysfunction, research is needed to determine new evaluation and cardiopulmonary training regimens emphasizing upper extremity activities. The primary goal of evaluation of cardiopulmonary response to specific amounts of exercise is to avoid unnecessary secondary cardiac and pulmonary complications resulting from overexertion. In the very old it is common to find patients who require basic cardiac conditioning before other physical therapy procedures can be safely administered.

REFERENCES

1. Brody SJ: The graying of America. Hospitals 54:63–66, 123, 1980.
2. Bassey EJ: Age, inactivity and some physiological responses to exercise. Gerontology 24:66–67, 1978.
3. Clarke HH: Exercise and aging. Physical Fitness Res Digest, Ser 7, no 2, April 1977.
4. Shephard RJ: Activity patterns of the elderly. In: Physical Activity and Aging, Year Book Medical Publishers, Chicago, 1978.
5. Sidney KH, Shephard RJ: Activity patterns of elderly men and women. J Gerontol 32:25–32, 1977.
6. Saltin B, Blomqvist B, Mitchel JH, et al: Response to submaximal and maximal exercise after bed rest and training. Circulation 38(Suppl 7), 1968.
7. Browse NL: The Physiology and Pathology of Bed Rest. Charles C Thomas, Springfield, Ill., 1965.
8. Graf RS: Rehabilitation during the acute and convalescent stages following myocardial infarction. In: Clinics in Physical Therapy: Cardiac Rehabilitation, ed. Amundsen LR. Churchill Livingston, New York, 1981.
9. Serfass RC: Exercise for the elderly: What are the benefits and how do we get started? In: Aging and Exercise, eds. Smith EL, Serfass RC. Enslow, Hillside, N.J., 1981.
10. Michel TH: Physiological effects of endurance training. In: Clinics in Physical Therapy: Cardiac Rehabilitation, ed. Amundsen LR. Churchill Livingstone, New York, 1981.
11. Karvonen MJ, Kentala E, Mustala O: The effects of training on heart rate. Ann Med Exp Biol Fenn 35:307–315, 1958.
12. Amundsen LR: Establishing activity and training levels for patients with ischemic heart disease. Phys Ther 59:754–758, 1979.
13. Carter CL: Cardiac rehabilitation of outpatients during the recovery stage following myocardial infarction. In: Clinics in Physical Therapy: Cardiac Rehabilitation, ed. Amundsen LR. Churchill Livingstone, New York, 1981.
14. Harris R: Cardiovascular system in rehabilitation of the elderly. NY State J Med 74:972–975, 1974.
15. Shepard RJ: Cardiovascular limitations in the aged. In: Exercise and Aging, eds. Smith EL, Serfass RC. Enslow, Hillside, N.J., 1981.
16. Fitts RH: Aging and skeletal muscle. In: Exercise and Aging, eds. Smith EL, Serfass RC. Enslow, Hillside, N.J., 1981.
17. Smith EL, Sempos CT, Purvis RW: Bone mass and strength decline with age. In: Exercise and Aging, eds. Smith EL, Serfass RC. Enslow, Hillside, N.J., 1981.
18. Reddan WG: Respiratory system and aging. In: Exercise and Aging, eds. Smith EL, Serfass RC. Enslow, Hillside, N.J., 1981.
19. de Vries HA: Physiological effects of an exercise training regimen upon men aged 52 to 88. J Gerontol 25:325–336, 1970.
20. Adams GM, de Vries HA: Physiological effects of an exercise training regimen upon women aged 52 to 79. J Gerontol 28:50–55, 1973.
21. Sidney KH, Shephard RJ, Harrison JE: Endurance training and body composition of the elderly. Am J Clin Nutr 30:326–333, 1977.
22. Barry AJ, Daly JW, Pruett ED, et al: The effects of physical conditioning on older individuals. I. Work capacity, circulatory-respiratory function, and work electrocardiogram. J Gerontol 21:182–191, 1966.
23. Suominen H, Heikkinen E, Liesen H, et al: Effects of 8 weeks' endurance training on

skeletal muscle metabolism in 56–70 year-old sedentary men. Eur J Appl Physiol 37:173–180, 1977.

24. Amundsen LR: Assessing exercise tolerance: A review. Phys Ther 59:534–537, 1979.
25. Amundsen LR, Nielsen DH: Normal and abnormal cardiovascular responses to acute physical exercise. In: Clinics in Physical Therapy: Cardiac Rehabilitation, ed. Amundsen LR. Churchill Livingstone, New York, 1981.
26. Shephard RJ: Gross changes in form and function. In: Physical Activity and Aging, Year Book Medical Publishers, Chicago, 1978.
27. Astrand P-O, Rodahl K: Textbook of Work Physiology, McGraw-Hill, New York, 1977.
28. Bates B: Pressures and Pulses: Arterial and venous. In: A Guide to Physical Examination. Lippincott, Philadelphia, 1979.
29. Schoneberger MB, Schoneberger B, Lundsford BR: Chart review and physical assessment prior to exercise. In: Clinics in Physical Therapy: Cardiac Rehabilitation, ed. Amundsen LR. Churchill Livingstone, New York, 1981.
30. Rowell LB: Human cardiovascular responses to exercise. In: Exercise and the Heart: Guidelines for Exercise Programs, ed. Morse RL. Charles C Thomas, Springfield, Ill., 1972.
31. Denolin H, Messin R, Degre S: Testing of the working capacity of cardiac patients. In: Physical Activity and the Heart, ed. Karvonen MJ and Barry AJ. Charles C Thomas, Springfield, Ill., 1967.
32. Jones NL, Campbell EJM, Edwards RHT, et al: Physiology of exercise. In: Clinical Exercise Testing. Saunders, Philadelphia, 1975.
33. American College of Sports Medicine: Guidelines for Graded Exercise Testing and Exercise Prescription. Lea & Febiger, Philadelphia, 1975.
34. Carlsten A, Grimby G: Effects of exercise on the central circulation. In: The Circulatory Response to Muscular Exercise in Man. Charles C Thomas, Springfield, Ill., 1966.
35. Naughton J, Haider R: Methods of exercise testing. In: Exercise Testing and Exercise Training in Coronary Heart Disease, ed. Naughton J, Hellerstein HK. Academic, New York, 1973.
36. Hellerstein NK, Hirsch EL, Ader R, et al: Principles of exercise prescription for normals and cardiac subjects. In: Exercise Testing and Exercise Training in Coronary Heart Disease, eds. Naughton J, Hellerstein H, Mohler IC. Academic, New York, 1973.
37. Anderson KL, Shephard RJ, Denolin H, et al: Techniques for collection and evaluation of cardiovascular and respiratory data during exercise. In: Fundamentals of Exercise Testing. World Health Organization, Geneva, 1971.
38. Physiological measurements and indices. In: Fitness, Health and Work Capacity: International Standards for Assessment, ed. Larson L. Macmillan, New York, 1973.
39. Haskell WL: Design and implementation of cardiac conditioning programs. In: Rehabilitation of the Coronary Patient. Wiley, New York, 1978.
40. Hellerstein HK, Franklin BA: Exercise testing and prescription. In: Rehabilitation of the Coronary Patient. Wiley, New York, 1978.
41. Nielsen DH, Amundsen LR: Exercise physiology: An overview with emphasis on aerobic capacity and energy cost. In: Clinics in Physical Therapy: Cardiac Rehabilitation, ed. Amundsen LR. Churchill Livingstone, New York, 1981.
42. McAllister RG, Lowenthal SL: Progressive exercise tolerance testing. In: Clinics in Physical Therapy: Cardiac Rehabilitation, ed. Amundsen LE. Churchill Livingstone, New York, 1981.
43. Sidney KH, Shephard RJ: Maximum and submaximum exercise tests in men and

women in the seventh, eighth, and ninth decades of life. J Appl Physiol 43:280–287, 1977.

44. Nielsen DH, Gerleman DG, Amundsen LR, et al: Clinical determination of energy cost and walking velocity via stopwatch or speedometer cane and conversion graphs. Phys Ther 62:591–596, 1982.

45. Parachek JF, King L: Parachek Geriatric Rating Scale. Greenroom Publishing, Scottsdale, Ariz., 1976.

46. Jette AM, Branch LG: The Framingham Study: II. Physical disability among the aging. Am J Public Health 71:1211–1216, 1981.

47. Jackson O: Functional assessment of the aged. Allied Hlth Behav Sci 2:47–59, 1980.

48. Lawton EB: Activities of Daily Living Test: Geriatric Considerations. Phys Occup Ther Geriatrics 1:11–20, 1980.

49. Mahoney FI, Barthel DW: Functional evaluation: The Barthel Index. Md State Med J 14:61–65, 1965.

50. Dinnerstein AJ, Lowenthal M, Dexter M: Evaluation of a rating scale of ability in Activities of Daily Living. Arch Phys Med Rehabil 46:579–584, 1965.

51. Aniansson A, Rundgrin A, Sperling L: Evaluation of functional capacity in activities of daily living in 70-year-old men and women. Scand J Rehabil Med 12:145–154, 1980.

52. Kottke FJ, Kubicek WG, Olson ME, et al: Five stage test of cardiac performance during occupational activity. Arch Phys Med Rehabil 43:228–234, 1962.

53. de Vries HA: Physiological effects of an exercise training regimen upon men aged 52–88. J Gerontol 25:325–336, 1970.

54. Adams GM, de Vries HA: Physiological effects of an exercise training regimen upon women aged 52 to 79. J Gerontol 28:50–55, 1973.

55. Sidney KH, Shephard RJ, Harrison JE: Endurance training and body composition of the elderly. Am J Clin Nutr 30:326–333, 1977.

56. Barry AJ, Daly JW, Pruett ED, et al: The effects of physical conditioning on older individuals. I. Work capacity, circulatory–respiratory function, and work electrocardiogram. J Gerontol 21:182–191, 1966.

57. Smith EL: Age: The interaction of nature and nurture. In: Exercise and Aging The Scientific Basis, eds. Smith EL, Serfass RC. Enslow, Hillside, N.J., 1981.

58. Sidney KH: Cardiovascular benefits of physical activity in the exercising aged. In: Exercise and Aging The Scientific Basis, eds. Smith EL, Serfass RC. Enslow, Hillside, N.J., 1981.

59. Sidney KH, Shephard RJ: Frequency and intensity of exercise training for elderly subjects. Med Sci Sports 10(2):125–131, 1978.

60. de Vries, HA: Prescription of exercise for older men from telemetered exercise heart rate data. Geriatrics 26:102–111, April 1971.

61. Morse CE, Smith EL: Physical activity programming for the aged. In: Exercise and Aging: The Scientific Basis, eds. Smith, EL, Serfass RC. Enslow, Hillside, N.J., 1981.

62. Activities Which Require a MET Level in the Cardiac Rehabilitation Program. Department of Physical Medicine, St. Joseph Mercy Hospital, Ann Arbor, 1972.

63. Greer M, Weber T, Dimick S, et al: Physiological responses to low-intensity cardiac rehabilitation exercises. Phys Ther 60:1146–1151, 1980.

64. Weise RA, Karpovich PV: Energy cost of exercises for convalescents. Arch Phys Med 28:447–454, 1947.

65. Fletcher GF, Cantwell JD, Watt EW: Oxygen consumption and hemodynamic response of exercises used in training of patients with recent myocardial infarction. Circulation 60:140–144, 1979.

66. Kellerman JJ, Ben-Ari E, Chayet M, et al: Cardiocirculatory response to different types of training in patients with angina pectoris. Cardiology 62:218–231, 1977.
67. Amundsen LR, Takahashi M, Carter CA, et al: Energy cost of rehabilitation calisthenics. Phys Ther 59:855–858, 1979.
68. Fleischaker KJ, Gower MA, Canafax LM, et al: Case Study: Rehabilitation following a myocardial infarction, with a sample program. In: Clinics in Physical Therapy. Cardiac Rehabilitation, ed. Amundsen LR. Churchill Livingstone, New York, 1981.
69. Lerman J, Bruce RA, Sivarajan E, et al: Low level dynamic exercises for earlier cardiac rehabilitation. Aerobic and hemodynamic responses. Arch Phys Med Rehabil 57:355–360, 1976.
70. David JA, Convertino VA: A comparison of heart rate methods for predicting endurance training intensity. Med Sci Sports 7:295–298, 1975.
71. Cassel J, Heyden SH, Bartel AG, et al: Occupational and physical activity and coronary heart disease. Arch Int Med 128:920–928, 1971.
72. Spielberger CD, Gorsuch RL, Lushene RE: The State–Trait Anxiety Inventory (STAI), test manual for Form X. Consulting Psychologists Press, Palo Alto, 1968.
73. Smith EL, Reddan W, Smith PE: Physical activity and calcium modalities for bone mineral increase in aged women. Med Sci Sports 13:60–64, 1981.

9 Functional Evaluation of the Elderly

Osa Jackson
Rosalie H. Lang

Applied gerontology takes didactic concepts and research findings out of the laboratory and uses them to enable functional evaluation to be the starting point of effective rehabilitation for the elderly. Functional evaluation assures a data base for this population, and for each individual within the population, that supports development of a comprehensive, rational, and efficient process of rehabilitation. The goal is maximum self-care, enhancing the possibility of an improved quality of life for patients limited by age and disability.

A good data base will also help us to know more about the financial abilities of the healthy elderly as well as the characteristic functional abilities of the frail at risk of institutionalization. We need to understand what enables independent living in the community—in order to develop realistic plans of care for the disabled. The overall result will be the creation of an organization, process, and philosophy of care that acknowledges the unique needs and functional capacities of the elderly as a group and of each individual.

Evaluation/assessment of the aged patient requires a clear definition of the term rehabilitation and an understanding of the need for the primary emphasis to be placed on functional ability rather than on diagnostic labels. A discussion of the important interrelationship between activities of daily living (ADL) and mental health will be presented as the justification for the need for a circle of care for the elderly. As a physical therapist, how do you fit into the circle of care? How do the activities of the other providers of care in your community (hospital, short-term rehabilitation, long-term rehabilitation, nursing home, home care, adult day care, respite care, meals on wheels, homemaker and chore services) affect the potential effectiveness of your efforts? How can the organization and approach of

Ms. Lang's research supported by Administration on Aging grant 90–A–1618.

institutional care affect the outcome of rehabilitation? Why is it that the majority of the elderly prefer and do better in a home-based rehabilitation program? Are home-based rehabilitation programs realistic as an alternative to residential/institutional rehabilitation? What are the major modifications needed? It is only with an understanding of the potential client and the total environment in which you are working that it is useful to begin to examine the actual details of the evaluation process. If basic premises about the patient population are not accurate or if the environment in which you are working does not support the intended outcome of your efforts (improving self-care capacity and quality of life for the aged patient), the physical therapist cannot expect to see improvements in functional capacity in the elderly patient.

The elderly may come to rehabilitation after a stroke, cardiovascular problem, orthopedic problem, or a combination of problems or as a result of a disruption in self-care capacity stemming from chronic degenerative disabilities accumulating over time. The elderly cannot be squeezed into a rehabilitation model or program based on the evaluation/treatment approaches used for the middle-aged population. This chapter presents a discussion of a model rehabilitation program or system incorporating a record-keeping system designed for the multiple functional problems commonly seen in the elderly. A model for in-depth ADL evaluation and ongoing monitoring of progress as it relates to self-care capacity also is presented. The basic premise of this chapter is that the elderly are a special population requiring a special philosophy and process of rehabilitation and physical therapy if they are to achieve their full potential.

THE ELDERLY—A POPULATION WITH INTENSIVE REHABILITATION NEEDS

The 1975 report from the United States Federal Commission on Chronic Illness[1] estimated a rate of 4402 chronic diseases per 1000 people 65 years of age and older, compared to 407 chronic diseases per 1000 people under the age of 16. It has been noted that it is only when functioning in day-to-day activities is affected that chronic illness becomes a matter of both public and private concern.[2] For example, a household survey[3] of a Rhode Island population in 1975 noted that 66.7 percent of the respondents age 65 and older suffered from a "longstanding condition" but that only 34.6 percent reported that it resulted in "some limitations in major activities." It is true that with advanced age there is increased incidence of chronic illness and disability, but it is a very small percentage of the elderly who require special, formal services.

In order to begin to examine the evaluation procedures that help to define the scope of the needed services, activities of daily living (ADL) will be defined as "all activities necessary during an ordinary day from waking up in the morning until going to sleep at night."[4] If it is possible to define the normal range of functional capabilities for the healthy and frail elderly, it will then be possible to begin to modify evaluation procedures to gain a better measure of the functional capacity of each elderly disabled patient. With realistic age norms, it is also possible to create increasingly appropriate restorative programs of care. The goal is to work to remove the age bias that now exists in evaluation of the aged as possible candidates for rehabilitation care, including the biases within the field of physical therapy. Increasingly targeted evaluation procedures will facilitate independence and active lives for the aged, an outcome beneficial to society and the elderly individual. A more important byproduct is that such procedures will make it possible to maintain independence among the healthy and better support frail elderly through environmental planning and modifications (e.g., housing design, kitchen organization).

The review of normative research findings in ADL capacity among the healthy and at risk elderly will be divided as follows: basal ADL (upper extremity function, hygiene, and dressing); function in the kitchen (pronation, supination, and reach); mobility (standing from a seated position in a chair, maintaining a comfortable walking speed, climbing steps); gross mobility; common physical activities; and social disability (housekeeping, transportation, socialization, food preparation, and grocery shopping).

Basal ADL

The functional capacity of the upper extremities is closely tied to basal activities of daily living (upper extremity function, hygiene, and dressing). Since upper extremity strength and its functional use seems to be less affected by advanced aging than strength of the lower extremities, the basal ADL appears to change least with age.[5] In spite of this fact the Framingham Disability Study found that the average healthy 75 to 84-year-old is likely to need more help to perform all basal ADLs except eating than persons 55 to 64. However, over 90 percent of the 75 to 84-year-olds were still independent in all basal ADLs. Women in the study were also more likely to require help with basal ADLs than men.[6] The Framingham Disability Study examined a population that is slightly less disabled than the average older person in the United States because of a higher-than-average socioeconomic status and longstanding selective participation in the study (nearly 30 years) of the population studied. A comparison with Branch's 1976 Massachusetts Elders Survey of noninstitutionalized elderly confirms the finding that the Framingham group was slightly less disabled than the norm.[7]

The test for upper extremity mobility used four tasks (reach for opposite big toe, grasp earlobe on opposite side with arm in front of head, grasp earlobe on opposite side with arm behind head, and fit hand between buttock and seat). The only task that the average 70-year-old tested had any difficulty with was the reach for the opposite big toe.[8] In this study 7.3 percent of the men and 5.5 percent of the women were not able or were able only with difficulty to reach their opposite big toe. This movement involves the integrated function of the upper extremity with the pelvis and lower extremity. If the big toe reach cannot be performed, there will be functional problems with dressing and pedicure. The need for assistive devices to compensate for the loss of integrated upper and lower extremity motion in the elderly is well documented.[9]

In order to facilitate improvement in basal ADL tasks, consider a review of the normative age-related changes in the component motions that has been made.[10] As compared to 20 to 30-year-olds, the average 70-year-old tested had no difference in strength of key grip or in endurance of the transversal volar grip. The lack of change in the key grip from young to old may be associated with the frequent use of this movement in ADL (e.g., handling keys, faucet handles, etc.). It was noted that there was a decrease in muscle coordination and strength of the transversal volar grip, visible in functional activities (e.g., handling an electric plug) for 70-year-old women, whose dexterity was found to be poorer than that of 70-year-old men at this task.[8] Researchers show a consensus in finding a decrease of hand strength in older men—35 to 43 percent between ages 25 and 74.[11, 12] Asmussen[13] found a decrease in the strength of the transversal volar grip of 23 percent in men from age 25 to age 65. In women overall, the loss of strength noted was less than for men. It appears that as the elderly lose strength in the transversal volar grip there is an increase in the submaximal endurance of this movement. Functionally, this may mean that there is a normal compensation in endurance for the decrease in strength. The compensation is noted more in women than in men.

Functional Kitchen Activities

Carroll developed tests for pronation and supination as a part of a quantitative test of upper-extremity function.[14] Along with a reach test, these tests were used to examine the normative levels of function related to basic eating and food preparation activities. Pouring water from a jug to a glass was used to test forearm pronation in a power and precision activity. The jug contained 1 liter of water. Pronation and supination of the forearm were tested in a precision activity by having subjects pour water from one glass to another and back again. It was found that among elderly 2.3 percent of the men and 1.8 percent of the women had difficulty in carrying out one or more of the tasks involved in the water-pouring test. The subjects who experienced difficulty were noted to have some locomotor dysfunctions and could not be classified as healthy.[8]

Upper-extremity reach was tested by having subjects lift a glass and a 1-kg packet onto shelves 140 to 180 cm high. The shelves were mounted above a cupboard 60 cm deep and 90 cm high, simulating a kitchen counter. It was found that 1.1 percent of the men and 6.9 percent of the women were not able to lift the glass and the weight to the shelf 180 cm high. There was an equal number of participants who could perform this task only with difficulty. With advanced age there is an associated decrease in height. It must be noted that even young women 158 cm tall or shorter have similar difficulty lifting a glass and a 1-kg packet to a shelf 180 cm high. Other causes that complicated the execution of the task were locomotor/neurologic problems or positional vertigo (head/neck extension). In the average elderly population living independently in the community, there appears to be enough difficulty with high reach to warrant systematic modifications of kitchen organization and design.

Mobility

The three components examined in this category are rising from a chair (seated position), walking speed (as it relates to pedestrian activity), and climbing steps (as it relates to use of public transportation). To rise from a seated position in a chair may require the assistance of the upper extremities. Sperling found no significant differences in strength of elbow extension between 70-year-old subjects and younger subjects.[10] This finding would imply that most elderly persons, if there is no pathology involving the upper extremities, can assist themselves in coming to a standing position *if arm rests are available.* Since lower-extremity function for this task is often decreased, furniture design can directly compensate for the age-related losses in the ability to rise from a chair.

For the walking test, subjects were asked to walk 30 meters unassisted (the distance across an average urban street). The increased interest in examining walking speed in the elderly is the result of the increasing rate of traffic accidents involving the elderly as pedestrians. The elderly on average walk slower than the speed defined as safe for crossing at traffic signals (1.4 meters/second). In a study of Swedish pedestrians, the elderly averaged a speed of 0.9 m/sec for normal walking, 1.1 m/sec for "hurrying," and only 1.3 m/sec if they were trying to catch a bus.[15] These research findings concur with the work of Lautso, who found that the average walking speed for the aged was 1.07 m/sec.[16] The aged have been noted to have major gait changes,[17, 18] and under stress elderly women particularly develop postural sway.[19] It was also noted that older men walk faster than older women; slower-walking men tended to be less physically active in leisure activities (no such correlation for women). The slowest-walking men and women were commonly dependent on a cane and often also had some upper-extremity problems or arthritis. It was found that walking speed correlated with height (taller persons tended to walk faster) but not with weight.[10]

As a person ages, ability to drive a car safely decreases. The elderly become increasingly dependent on various means of public transportation, all involving some stepping into and out of the vehicle (bus, train). In the step test, all 70-year-old subjects could master steps of 10, 20, and 30 cm without handrails. All 70-year-old men and women tested could climb up and down a 40-cm step with a handrail. For a 40-cm step with no handrail, 4 of the men and 23 of women could not step up and 5 men and 10 women could not step down. At a 50-cm step nearly all men and women could manage, some with difficulty, with a rail, but without a handrail 10 men and 71 women could not get up and 9 men and 34 women could not get down. Women appeared to have more difficulties than men with the step test. Inverse correlations were found for 70-year-old women between step height and weight with no railing for both going up the step and coming down (no such correlation for men). For elderly women a correlation was also noted between maximum step height up/down without a railing and maximum dynamic muscle strength of the quadriceps muscle at the probable contractile velocity used when climbing up or down steps and isometric muscle strength at 60° and 90° knee angles. In both sexes a correlation was noted between maximum step height up/down and walking speed.[8]

The functional implication is that the average elderly person can manage to go up and down steps of up to 30 cm with no railing, 40 cm if a railing is available. A public transportation vehicle that has a step of 50 cm or higher, with or without a railing, represents a difficult obstacle, especially for elderly women. It has been found that older women (75+) seem to have less control stepping down than older men and younger women.[20] Given these basic data, it is crucial that we work to facilitate modifications in step height in all types of public transportation. A purchase of a poorly designed bus can result in 10 years of difficulty for the aged on that bus line until the bus wears out (for trains the lifespan of a car may be up to 40 years). Yet moderate adaptation of step height and the use of handrails in public transportation can facilitate independence for the elderly by increasing their ability to be mobile.

Gross Mobility

The Rosow-Breslau test was used to examine the ability of the elderly, 55 to 84 years of age, to perform heavy housework, walk 0.5 miles (0.8 km) and climb stairs.[21] The results noted in the Framingham Disability Study demonstrate that a substantially smaller number of subjects are able to perform these activities than can perform all basal ADL. Only 50 percent of the oldest group (75 to 84 years old) were able to perform heavy household work as compared to 79 percent of the 55 to 64-year-old group; 77 percent of the oldest group were able to walk 0.5 miles, compared to 96 percent of the 55 to 64-year-old group; and 85 percent of the oldest group were able to climb stairs, compared to 97 percent of the younger group.

It is relevant that over three fourths of those 75 to 84 years old report that they are still able to climb stairs and walk at least 0.5 miles (but reporter reliability needs to be studied by actual task execution). Overall, women report performing more poorly than men, especially as age increases, but again this may not be realistic—actual task execution must be studied.[6]

These findings point up the need for supportive services to assist the elderly with heavy household work. As the maintenance of a home gradually deteriorates, the mental health of the high risk elderly may be affected, which could become a contributing cause of depression. A key to rehabilitation is that supportive intervention for heavy housework, if it is a task valued by the patient, may greatly improve the person's mental health and outlook.

Physical Activities Profile

In the Framingham Disability Study, 55 to 84-year-olds were asked to describe their ability to perform nine physical activities (extending arms below shoulders, extending arms above shoulders, lifting weight under 10 pounds/4 kg, sitting for 1+ hours, standing for 15+ minutes, moving large objects, lifting weight over 10 pounds/4 kg, stooping/crouching/kneeling). It was found that 80 percent of the total sample were able to extend their arms in both directions, lift weights under 10 pounds/4 kg, sit for long periods, and hold small objects without difficulty. The proportion of elderly performing these five activities without difficulty decreased with advancing age (74 percent of the oldest members reported no difficulty). A notably smaller percentage of women than men stated that they could perform these five activities without difficulty. Among the group 75 to 84 years of age, only 67 percent of the women, compared to 90 percent of the men, reported no difficulty in lifting weights under 10 pounds/4 kg (largest age-specific gender difference).

The remaining physical activities are highly significant for housekeeping, food preparation, use of public transportation, and grocery shopping, and they appear to be greatly affected by advanced age. Only 73 percent of the total sample reported that they experienced no difficulty standing longer than 15 minutes, and among the oldest group (75 to 84) only 58 percent of the women and 67 percent of the men reported no difficulty.* The loss or perceived loss of this physical ability increasingly limits the very old in their use of public transportation and in doing their own grocery shopping, since it becomes difficult to ensure a supportive environment (e.g., seats, benches, or chairs to rest on).

Some 66 percent of the total sample noted they could perform the task of moving large objects without difficulty. In the oldest group (75 to 85) only 48 percent of the women but 80 percent of the men felt that they could still perform this task without difficulty. Functionally, the loss or perceived loss of the ability to move large objects has direct impact on home maintenance and creates special problems for the older single or widowed woman.

Some 65 percent of the total sample ages 55 to 84 reported achieving the task of lifting weights over 10 pounds without difficulty. For 55 to 64-year-olds only 59 percent of the women could complete the task successfully, at 65 to 74 years of age only 55 percent and for the oldest group (75 to 84) the success figure was 34 percent. The men reported less difficulty, with 87 percent of the 55 to 64-year-olds successful, 85 percent of the 65 to 74-year-olds, and 72 percent of the 75 to 84-year-olds.

Lastly, only 59 percent of the total sample reported completing the physical activity of stooping/crouching/kneeling without difficulty. The same trend was noted as was seen for lifting weights over 10 pounds—the men reported greater success at all ages than the women, and a gradual decrease in ability noted for both sexes with advanced age. There are major functional implications for the finding that only 38 percent of the women and 59 percent of the men 75 to 84 years of age reported successful completion of this movement.[12]

Social Disability

The pivotal tasks affecting a person's ability to live independently are housekeeping, transportation, social interaction, food preparation, and grocery shopping. Studies of the capacity of elderly persons for physical activities such as standing for longer periods of time, lifting objects heavier than 10 pounds/4 kg, and kneeling indicate that with advancing age there is increasing difficulty in performing the basic social tasks needed for independent living in the community. In the FDS only 6 percent of the total sample of 55 to 84-year-olds interviewed had unmet needs in one or more of the social tasks; however, one fourth of the elderly

---

* It must again be noted that the subjects in the Framingham Disability Study (FDS) tended to be healthier than the average older person in the United States. Shanas estimates that 12 of every 100 elderly (65 and older) have a major incapacity index, but the FDS only found 7 percent.[22] This discrepancy may be partly explained by the presence of persons over age 85 in the Shanas study; all subjects in the FDS were 84 years of age or younger.

were *at risk* of developing unmet needs in one or more of the social tasks.

Housekeeping and transportation were the two social tasks with the highest prevalence of unmet need or risk of unmet need. It was found that three times as many 75 to 84-year-olds as 55 to 64-year-olds had unmet needs (but this was still only 12 percent of the oldest group). Housekeeping tasks involved the greatest reported difficulty; 15 percent of 55 to 64-year-olds and 25 percent of the oldest group experienced difficulty with housekeeping. Women were found to have more unmet needs for housekeeping and transportation than the men. Housekeeping—the ability to keep the home orderly, neat, and clean by one's individual standards—and transportation to carry out basic tasks for independence and meaningful survival in the community are pivotal to the mental as well as physical well-being of the elderly. The loss of the ability to perform these social tasks can contribute to depression and related physical dysfunction due to stress.

It is estimated that in the year 2000 20 percent of the United States population will be over age 65 and half of this group will be 75 years of age or older.[23] Physical capacity to perform tasks involving mobility and the basic survival activities for independent living in the community decreases with increasing age. The research documenting the functional abilities of the elderly as a group, particularly the very old (85+), is only in the beginning stages. The data that already exist (FDS, Shanas, Aniansson, etc.) point to the increasing need to modify the environment to facilitate independent living for the elderly and especially the very old. Should not the hospital, clinic, and nursing home provide the basic environmental and organizational modifications to support maximum function for elderly with rehabilitation potential? What is the role of the health care providers (rehabilitation team) in facilitating the postfacility adjustment of the disabled elderly in the community in light of their special needs (e.g., housekeeping, transportation) during the early weeks of home care? The special functional needs of some elderly mandate examination of the evaluation procedures used for rehabilitation and discharge planning to ensure that they incorporate the potential areas of high risk unique to the very old.

REHABILITATION FOR THE ELDERLY—A SPECIAL APPROACH

The cost of premature institutionalization of the elderly is staggering. Modifications in the total rehabilitation process to incorporate the special functional characteristics of the elderly population will allow a greater number of elderly to reach a higher level of self-care capacity. Barry indicates that there is potential for better mental and physical health among older people if their independence can be supported.[24] The ability to perform ADL affects mental health, and the description or diagnosis generally does not predict the functional capacity of the client mentally or physically. A discussion of interrelationship of function, diagnosis, and mental health is used here as the basis for the development of the concept of total care or a circle of care for the elderly. The need for a comprehensive approach to care of the disabled elderly forces us to examine the components of care, their interrelationship, the organization and the role of home-based care, and its unique contribution to the social and emotional well-being of the aged.

Independent Living Rehabilitation

The elderly are an increasingly visible group who are conscious of the positive potential of rehabilitation. Yet the disabled elderly have been unserved or underserved by all members of the rehabilitation team.[25,26] This lack was largely related to the original definition of rehabilitation, which was based on the potential for return to employment, since the majority of persons needing rehabilitation were of employable age. The demographics are changing, and the elderly population will increase in percentage of the total population for many years. The advent of independent living rehabilitation (ILR) can be seen as a beginning toward promoting self-help, consumer involvement, and prevention of premature institutional care for the disabled elderly. A contemporary definition of ILR is as follows:[27]

> [ILR requires] control over one's life based on the choice of acceptable options that minimize reliance on others in making decisions and in performing everyday activities. This includes managing one's own affairs; participating in day-to-day life in the community; fulfilling a range of social roles; and making decisions that lead to self determination and the minimization of psychological or physical dependence on others. Independence is a relative concept, which may be defined personally by each individual.

Statistics show that independent living is an issue of grave concern as a part of advanced aging:

- 17 percent of the elderly were "unable to carry on their major activities;"[28]
- The baseline average is one disabled in ten Americans, but for those over age 65 it is one in three;[29]
- 20 percent of older people 65 to 74 years of age and almost 42.5 percent of those over 75 have "substantial and severe limitations in physical and emotional performance;"[30]
- 11.5 percent of disabled 65 to 74 years of age need mobility or personal care assistance for independent living, and the percentage increases to 25.8 percent for those over 75 years of age.[30]

The elderly are underrepresented as rehabilitation clients, particularly in light of their proportion in the population of persons with disabilities.[31]

ILR is an approach that can work for the elderly disabled because older disabled persons require the same basic services as other disabled, although they may require them for a longer period of time. Among the services that are crucial (owing to the unique physical, emotional, and functional abilities among the elderly) are the following:

1. Group counseling, with special emphasis on motivation, reality, and support groups;
2. Mobility assistance—e.g., shopping help, transportation, and adaptive training for those with failing sight;
3. Homemaker services—e.g., attendant care, meals on wheels, "Friendly Visitor," etc.;
4. Information, referral, and advocacy;
5. Coordination among the various agencies, programs, and services–service system management on behalf of individual elderly to assure care appropriate to their functional status.

In 1978 the Rehabilitation Services Administration (RSA) funded five ILR demonstration projects in the United States, but only one of the projects included the aged as part of the target population.[27] The emphasis needs to change—the Urban Institute estimates that in 1975 there were 10 million noninstitutionalized severely disabled persons in the United States, and 4 million of them (40 percent) were 65 years old or older.[29]

ILR should emphasize restoration of independent living skills during short- or long-term-facility care for acute illness. Driscoll et al. noted that if the elderly can avoid taking on the role of the "good patient," they then avoid the need to lose this dependency and the lack of self-directed behavior at the moment of discharge to the community.[32] This may be an unrealistic expectation, however, in view of the dependency-creating characteristics of institutional care.

ADL—Functional Versus Diagnostic Emphasis

In the presence of unlimited fiscal resources, health care for the elderly can be built on a crisis intervention, diagnostic model. Even with unlimited resources, given the chronic nature of most disabilities, crisis care could never provide the most effective model of improved function as the goal. The reality of health care today is that there are limited fiscal and manpower resources available, in light of which it is crucial that any intervention beyond the life-or-death or emergency situation be focused on facilitating the elderly clients' independence and overall well-being. For the disabled elderly, it is crucial to build from two concepts that have been shown to affect their adjustment in any new situation: (1) what the person desires or values, and (2) the extent to which it is obtainable.

The joint interaction of these two factors is referred to by Reed and Ziegler as a person's "locus of desired control;" their research has shown substantial and reliable correlations between locus of desired control and psychologic adjustment.[33] The physical ability of the elderly to carry out the ADLs described in the previous section decreases gradually with advancing age. However, it is crucial to note that there is great variability among the elderly; the majority even in the oldest groups studied (75 to 84 years of age) were able to carry out the ADLs needed for independent living in the community.

When an elderly person has a stroke or a hip fracture there are no predictable functional changes. A stroke patient does not always lose the ability to perform an

ADL task. The loss of functional ability to perform an ADL task requires the identification of deficits concomitant with assessed visual/motor impairment. The significance of an organic or pathologic diagnostic label must be interpreted individually with each elderly person in order to identify the behavioral implications. That is, the "organic difficulties should be interpreted in terms of the patient's observable function."[34] Only if evaluation is done with a functional emphasis is it possible to help the client think in concrete *self-help* terms, such as, "I've had a stroke and I want to learn to get on and off the toilet—that is important to me." The alternative is to evaluate the aged as we do with the young, examining range of motion, strength, spasticity, and so on as the primary emphasis, which can only lead to a reinforcement of loss rather than self-help. The young tend to have more psychologic stamina and broader support networks thus the lack of functional emphasis does not impact as severely as for the aged. The process of care, not just the intended outcome, must support psychologic adjustment as part of rehabilitation of the functional losses. (NOTE: Use of range of motion, strength evaluation, etc. can and should be used once functional goals are identified to evaluate details of loss and to help one design a treatment program, but such factors should never be used as the primary approach.)

There are psychologic implications of the ability to perform ADLs, and a loss of such ability will result in a direct loss of self-esteem and perceived control.[35] *If the rehabilitation team and therefore the elderly disabled client can focus on self-care capacity as a starting point, the patient will begin to understand that the component skills of basal self-care are also the foundation skills of the ability for independent living.*

It has been noted that physical impairment, age, depression, and disorientation have a strong interrelationship.[36] Therefore with any loss in the ability to perform basal ADLs (temporary or permanent), the psychologic reaction must also be examined. If depression develops in response to a temporary or permanent loss, an evaluation of the extent of emotional reaction must be examined if realistic evaluation and plan of care are to be developed.

A person needs some mental clarity to relearn ADL;[37] however, with use of assessment tools with a functional emphasis (i.e., tools that give insight into how the individual learns and communicates) it is possible to improve functional status of elderly persons with major distortion of emotional and cognitive abilities.[38] Ultimately, the goal of independent living is achieved only by working with the whole person—physical and mental dysfunctions and the emotional and functional implications of those dysfunctions.

Circle of Care for the Disabled Elderly

The circle of care for the elderly consists of the full range of medical, social, and environmental services, including meals on wheels, chore services, housekeeping, home health (including in-home rehabilitation specialists), senior centers, adult day care, telephone reassurance, respite care, homes for the aged, nursing homes, rehabilitation centers, hospitals, and many others. For the disabled elderly who have had a major medical problem, the point of entry into the circle is usually the hospital. For the disabled elderly who have severe chronic degenerative disease, the point of entry may lie with any provider in the circle. The intent of a circle of care is to assure that once identified, the elderly client receives care, over time, appropriate to need and functional status and becomes a part of a preventive health maintenance effort. The fact that one fourth of the independent elderly over age 75 in the Framingham Disability Study were found to be at risk for problems related to social survival in the community should sensitize us to the precarious independence of the disabled elderly.

Interrelationship and intercommunication among components of the basic health and social service network are crucial for support of the maximum level of independent living among the elderly. Owing to the differences between young and old in psychologic and sociologic status and functional skills, the high-risk/frail elderly need the support of the entire network to remain in *their* preferred living environment, which is usually their own home. Implicit in the need for intercommunication among the network of providers who track and provide services to maintain health and independence is the need for longitudinal record-keeping with a problem-oriented focus. Such need is especially acute if the elderly client has any form of mental status decline.

Organization and management of care of the elderly disabled client must include respect for confidentiality and the client's own needs and desires concerning plans of care. One way of dealing with the decrease of physical capacity or mental status of the client is to have an independent evaluation process that will assist and enable implementation of flexible, dynamically changing plans of care for the frail or high-risk aged who because of their physical and/or mental status are unable to effectively coordinate the network of care they require to remain independent in the community (see the discussion of Model Approach—Rehabilitation for the Elderly, below).

If the elderly disabled do require hospital care, the quality of the experience can affect every other component within the circle of care. The hospital environment and program of care should support maximum independence and self-directed behavior in patients beyond life-or-death crisis, which should involve individual plans of care allowing for self-care in all areas where the patient is able to perform.

The philosophy of care within the hospital must clearly be defined from the emergency room and the recovery room to the patient's room. For the elderly, as for other age groups, the emergency room and the recovery room are situations in which staff are in charge and are doing things *for* the patient. Once the elderly patient is back in his or her own room, the hospital staff must reorient themselves and the patient to support a philosophy of independent and self-directed behavior. The work load of the nursing staff is affected by the intent of the care plan in effect for the patient. Basal ADLs must be the concern of nursing care both to reduce the work overload caused by an increasingly aged hospital population and to assure care that supports the dignity and choices of patients regardless of illness and disability. For example, incontinence is not a factor that contributes to staff work load if an adequate toileting policy is implemented; however, if there is inadequate staff and concomitantly a poor toileting policy, the nursing workload will increase, patient morale will decrease, and the overall rehabilitation outcome will be negatively affected.

It is probably true that to facilitate rehabilitation, especially in the acute hospital, staff levels must be above those required for acute care, since the partially mobile patient requires more and different types of care than a bedridden patient.[39] If this challenge can be met, the 80-year-old stroke patient, for example, may need a longer rehabilitation effort but will do as well as the younger stroke patient.[40]

If the level of functional disability but not age[40] relates to future placement, is a geriatric rehabilitation unit a positive step after acute hospital care? In a time of limited resources, the key to the effectiveness of a geriatric rehabilitation unit is the ability to pick patients who need the special benefits of such a unit. Hall noted that patients with a favorable diagnosis can make progress in any hospital setting as long as the basic medical and rehabilitation components are present,[41] but patients with unfavorable diagnoses need total environmental and organizational support in order to improve to desired levels of independence. Available research data indicate that bowel and bladder function, ability to walk, and mental status are the major predictors of rehabilitation outcome.[42] In a study of 76-year-old patients admitted to a geriatric rehabilitation unit, 20 percent went home, 28 percent to a home for the aged, and 52 percent to a nursing home; it is significant that age was not a predictor of rehabilitation outcome.[40]

The plan of care within an institutionally based geriatric rehabilitation program must take account of experience demonstrating that patients can be out of their own environment no more than 3 months and still be likely to reintegrate at the completion of rehabilitation.[43] It is essential not to distort or displace the informal support network available to the elderly patient if that informal network is to be available upon discharge. In fact, in rehabilitation of the elderly special efforts must be made to evaluate, orient, and train those within the informal network so that they can accept and support the patient at discharge, another reason for identifying clearly the intended outcome of rehabilitation (independent living) and helping all within the circle of care (patient, family, rehabilitation team) to focus on functional ability.

As a part of the evaluation procedures for a rehabilitation unit, the Barthel Index (or the modified Barthel Index) has received a lot of attention. The Barthel Index measures the degree of physical handicap regardless of the particular diagnostic designations. It is an accurate measure of the degree of physical impairment as it relates to basic ADL function. It is thus a screening tool that can describe overall functional capacity, physical function, decision making, and ability to fulfill usual or customary roles. The screening of a patient with the Barthel Index can lead to a referral for indepth ADL evaluation by physical or occupational therapists.[36]

Home care or home-based rehabilitation programs (using visiting physical therapists, occupational therapists or nurses, adult day care, etc.) is the part of the circle of care most sought by the majority of the elderly.[44] This fact may be related to how our needs for belonging, love, and esteem can better be met in the community than within the structure and process of institutional care.[45]

The current emphasis of reimbursement for care in institutions is based on the visible, tangible physical intervention and the ease for providers of facility-based intervention, but home-based rehabilitation programs offer special support by the very structure of care for the patient (own environment, familiarity) and by involvement of the informal network.

The home-care setting allows rehabilitation with an emphasis on the needs of the patient and an acceptance of the patient's preferred environment. For the rehabilitation team, home care allows the clinician to examine the interrelation and complexity of management of multiple problems (diagnostic and functional) involved in the care of the aged. It is not unusual to have a case history based on an isolated systems review that results in a problem list like the following:[46]

List 1—Medical
 1. Hearing impairment
    - Unable to hear normal speech tones
 2. Vision impairment
    - Difficulty seeing small print
    - Difficulty seeing distant objects
 3. Speech and language impairment
    - Relies on spouse to answer
 4. Respiration impairment
    - Shortness of breath with exertion
 5. Neuromuscular skeletal function impairment
    - Limited range of motion
    - Inability to manage some ADL
    - Poor coordination
 6. Circulation impairment
    - Edema in lower extremities
    - Occasional irregular heart beat
 7. Digestive function impairment
    - Anorexia
    - Some weight loss
 8. Dentition impairment
    - Ill-fitting dentures
 9. Bowel function impairment
    - Incontinence
    - Constipation
10. Urinary function impairment
    - Incontinent
    - Inability to empty bladder
11. Nutrition impairment
    - Lacks proper caloric intake
    - Improper feeding schedule
    - Lacks essential vitamins, minerals, and food groups.
12. Physical activity impairment
    - Sedentary lifestyle; lacks regular exercise

13. Therapeutic regimen noncompliance
     * Failed to return to ophthalmologist for postcataract lenses
14. Income—possible deficit
     * Noncompliance due to worry about bills

A problem-oriented approach coordinated with a home-care process facilitates the examination of the interrelation of function and diagnostic problems. Such an approach enables clinicians to direct limited time and resources to the cluster of services that can improve or facilitate maximum independence within a rehabilitation framework.

For example, in the sample case above, when the problems were studied and reorganized based on a functional approach, targets of intervention changed drastically:[46]

List 2—Functional Problems in Light of Medical and/or Social Problems
1. Social isolation
    * Overdependence on wife, who speaks for patient
2. Related medical
    * Bowel function impairment: incontinency, constipation
    * Urinary function impairment: incontinence, inability to fully empty bladder
    * Hearing impairment
    * Vision impairment
3. Nutrition/digestive
    * Anorexia
    * Lacks proper calorie and nutrient intake
    * Dentition (poorly fitting dentures)
    * Constipation—see problem
4. Mobility/ADL limitation
    Related medical
    * Respiration—shortness of breath
    * Circulation—edema, irregular heart beat
    * Neuromusculoskeletal—limited range of motion, balance/coordination
    See problem 2—vision impairment
5. Income
    * Vision impairment—failure to return for glasses after cataract surgery
    * Dentition—ill-fitting dentures

List 1 resulted in a plan of care that relied primarily on the nursing care of the home health agency, with physician oversight. List 2 includes all the medical problems identified in list 1, but it relates those problems to *loss of function*. Therefore a high priority was placed on the following:

Congregate meals program
Male companionship for the husband
Respite for the wife, who was giving total care

Financial counseling to facilitate purchase of glasses and attention to dentures
Attention to balance, coordination, breathing difficulties, and effective therapeutic exercise program

The medical problems required continuing physician oversight and collaboration with the home health agency, which worked on bowel and bladder control, diet control, and monitoring of respiration and circulation. However, the medical regimen took on goals for mobility and social interaction implicit in a rehabilitative framework.

Home care intervention must be focused on functional needs in order to preserve the precarious independent living situation of the disabled elderly; this focus *can* be cost effective.[47] The reality today is that the cost of all institutional care is increasing. The organization and process of care must be reexamined and modified—the care provided in many hospitals and nursing homes is not therapeutic and diminishes the independence of the disabled elderly. Yet in the wake of rising costs the U.S. Federal Health Care Policy strongly supports institutional based care. In 1977 the budget for facility care was 12.6 billion dollars, compared to 575 million dollars for Medicare and Medicaid ambulatory and home care services. It is necessary to modify national health policy if the physiologic, psychologic, and social needs of the aged are to be supported to enable independent living into very old age for as many as possible.[48]

Current policies and related systems of care do not acknowledge the increasing *risk* of functional changes with advanced age (e.g., ability to stand for 15+ minutes, lift 10 pounds/4 kg or heavier, kneel) and the risk of social disability (loss of ability to shop for groceries, prepare meals, and use public transportation). Identification of the risk is the first step in appropriate management of the range of problems. More research will be valuable to gain more precise understanding of this population and their needs, but the effectiveness of rehabilitation coupled with attention to environmental and organizational modification to support independence of the high-risk elderly through all components of the circle of care has been amply demonstrated.

MODEL APPROACH—REHABILITATION FOR THE ELDERLY

The elderly as a group sustain many physiologic, psychologic, and social losses as a part of the normal aging process. In spite of this, the majority of the elderly continue to maintain the basic functional skills needed for independent living in the community. Through research, patterns of functional loss (ADL and social) have been identified as common in the healthy elderly, and there are distinctive patterns defining elderly as being *at risk* of loss of basic functional skills necessary for independent living. When the elderly became disabled due to acute or chronic degenerative illness, it is necessary that rehabilitation and patient evaluation incorporate not only the current illness or disability but also any previous functional losses, temporary functional losses due to the current illness, and the risk of future ADL and social functional losses.

The Service Coordination System (SCS) provides a system of assessment that can enable continuity of care through information sharing among hospital, home care, and community providers, patient, and family. The SCS is a way to organize service delivery for the aged from the community (preliminary problems), hospital (crisis), home care (short-term restorative care), nursing home (long-term restorative care), and then back to the community. The structure of SCS provides a tracking and coordination capacity in support of high-risk elderly as they move through a complicated and fast-paced health care delivery system. As health and service systems become increasingly accommodated to the elderly, SCS will be needed only in the nonhospital environment; until that time, the elderly will require a coordination program such as SCS to integrate their service needs at each level of medical/social intervention.

The Client Screen

The potential client's first contact with SCS is through a screening process designed to target care intensively to those at risk of functional losses. The screen has various formats, depending on whether patients are self-referred, are referred by others, or are referred during hospital stay. It can be adapted to multiple settings.

The screening interview (by phone or in person) is standardized and can be carried out by relatively unskilled interviewers. The interviewer gathers information on all ADLs that affect survival in the community: communication/cognition—can patients communicate, can they remember (especially short-term memory); mobility/transfer; feeding; toileting—both volitional control and self-care; emotional state; and home situation—level of assistance available, level of social support.

It is significant that the emphasis of the screening process is self-care tasks and identification of task limitations. It seeks to determine what persons can or cannot do for themselves. It is a function screen.

The screen probes for short-term memory loss in a functional way. Patients are asked to describe the primary problem(s) and how the problem(s) affect their life and their ability to do what is important to them. At the end of the screening interview, patients are asked to review their primary problem(s) for the interviewer to assure accuracy. A person with significant and functional memory loss is likely not to be able to remember what was described the first time, even a few minutes earlier.

Since the organic brain syndromes (including senile dementia of the Alzheimer type) and depression mimicking senility are among the most significant predictors of institutionalization, *early* identification of short-term memory loss is crucial to a successful screening and intervention program. Equally important is the fact that for the person for whom memory loss is not a problem, the request to review the primary problem(s) to ensure that the interviewer understands them accurately will not be offensive. The screen is designed to assess the patient's capacity to function at home, either alone or with assistance.

For situations where the client is not self-referring, the screen elicits information that is especially important if the caller is the primary caretaker. The need may exist for assistance to the primary caretaker to enable the caretaker to continue in that role. The screen can identify supporter stress that unless relieved can lead to an institutional placement undesired by client and family.

If the client is referred by a hospital, other institution, or social agency, the screen is adapted to integrate standardized isolated medical data with functional data related to self-care, community networking, and client goals. *Throughout SCS, an effort is made to facilitate self-directed behavior in the client by the format and process of care.* It is only in this way that it is possible to motivate patients to work with commitment toward realizing their potential.

Client Orientation and Confidentiality

If the interview or referral indicates that the patient is experiencing functional problems and an assessment in depth is required, the client is given a brochure and letter describing the SCS. A consent form for basic information sharing among practitioners is also included. In this way the patient and family or significant others have time to review the documents and prepare questions or voice concerns. When the members of the assessment team (a rehabilitation nurse or physical or occupational therapist *and* a social worker) arrive, they can answer any questions about the SCS.

Rules governing staff conduct relative to confidentiality and disclosure of records must be prepared as part of the implementation of SCS. Staff training includes emphasis on informed consent and the importance of confidentiality.

A questionnaire (patient history—self-report) is also sent to the patient as

Do you experience any of the following:	Check No	Yes	When did it start?	What tasks does this keep you from doing?
Tired				
Unwell				
Weak				
Gain in weight				
Loss in weight				
Hoarseness				
Sore tongue				
Difficulty swallowing				
Headache				
Dizziness				
Noises in ears				
Belching				
Heartburn				

Fig. 9-1.   Excerpt from patient self-history chart.

part of the introductory packet. The assumption is made that most people, given a chance, want to take responsibility for their own lives and will do so if they can. The self-report gathers information from the patient about past and present illnesses, bed days in home and in hospital, and significant losses and includes a full checklist of symptoms (see Figure 9-1). The self-report form is presented in non-medical language and large print to facilitate elderly client participation. It communicates to the patient and family that "you are a participating partner in your care; you and your family have the best information about how you feel and what you are experiencing."

SCS by its format of information collection attempts to strengthen the independence of the client. Clients fill out the form at their own pace and have time to reflect on the questions asked. The self-report provides a valuable tool for cross-validation of client responses during the actual assessment and with the physician summary. The fact that a given client cannot or chooses not to complete the self-report is also a valuable datum. The goal of the patient self-history is to build a "locus of control," which is known to facilitate psychologic well-being.[33]

Assessment

The goal of the assessment procedure is to produce sufficient information to allow valid and reliable judgments about service needs. Potential services can be formal or informal, free or paid for, but they should match the needs of the patient/client at any given time. Decisions about service needs based solely on medical or social data in isolation from the other variables have at least some probability of being wrong. To be patient-effective and cost-effective, services must be appropriate to needs. An unneeded service, no matter how fine, may sap independence in the client and is always wasteful.

The core assessment has nine basic categories of data collection:

Socioeconomic data: Basic descriptive data to enable determination of financial eligibility for services, primary language, education, employment history, and source of referral.

History:
1. Directory of services/providers—A descriptive list of all services/providers used by the client, the date that client was last seen or services were last used, the types of services received, and the goal or purpose of those services (this directory allows SCS to build on the system already in place).
2. Family history—Family illness history and a brief examination of family interaction, identifying primary source of information during the assessment.
3. Self-history—A review of the self-report form to assure that the client understood the questions and to discuss the answers.

Risk factors: Nutrition, obesity, dentition, substance abuse (including smoking and alcohol).

Problem No.	Category	Specific Medication	Dose	Freq.	Route	Length/ Time	Half- Life
	Analgesics/ narcotics						
	Antacids						
	Antibiotics/ antiinfectives						
	Anticoagulants						
	Anticonvulsants						
	Antihypertensives						
	Bowel regulators						
	Bronchodilators						
	Cardiac regulators						
	Diuretics/ electrolytes						
	Insulin/ hypoglycemics						
	Sedatives barbiturates						

Fig. 9-2. Excerpt from medication review. Specify each medication by category. Include dose; frequency; route of administration; length of time on medication; and half-life. Data also requested: Does patient understand purpose and side effects of medication? Who were medication instructions given by? Medication No.? Date of original Rx? Date last filled? MD ordering? Pharmacy (see service directory)? Date terminated?

Medications: A special emphasis is given this segment (see Figure 9-2). A review is made of the 18 basic categories of medications, the client's use of over-the-counter and prescription drugs, the patient's understanding of the medications and their use, and patient compliance (including review of patient education about medication use). At the completion of the assessment a review is made of medication–medication and medication–food interactions, significant problems for the elderly.

Sensation, balance, and proprioception: A review to examine status—functional with compensation (if so, what type?), partial loss of function with compensation, full loss, date of onset, and whether gradual or sudden.

Musculoskeletal: A full review of functional range of motion (amount of joint motion needed for basic self-care tasks), if limited, a comparison of active and passive movements of affected joints, and a note of functional tasks affected.

[NOTE: The core assessment team is composed of a rehabilitation nurse or a PT/OT to ensure the ability to provide a functional emphasis to the initial evaluation. The assessment is not meant to replace the in-depth PT/OT evaluation that is ordered as more details are required (after the core team has reviewed the assessment, physician summary, and the patient's self-history).]

Activities of daily living (ADL):   A systematic review of the client's ability to do each of the following tasks, along with the amount and type of help needed (as applicable) and related health care status and mobility status as they relate to each ADL task:

1. Personal care (bathing, grooming, dressing eating/feeding);
2. Communication (spoken and instrumental—telephone, writing, electronic);
3. Excretory functions (bowel and bladder);
4. Mobility skills (transfers and ambulation).

Mental status: An assessment of subjective mental status (how person feels and relates to others) and objective mental status (competence to direct one's own life, to remember, to comprehend, to follow instructions, to calculate, to understand basic spatial relationships, and to behave within acceptable norms). The mental status assessment has a functional orientation and emphasizes all the primary component skills used in communication and teaching. It is designed to facilitate identification of any special therapeutic support necessary to increase the client's potential to participate in the plan of care. (For example, if a client were unable to copy a simple design, such as a pair of interlocking pentagons, how would you modify the process of teaching this patient to use a walker?)

Environmental: A review of support resources as well as constraints to independence, including a detailed survey of the physical environment and economic status. The family and significant others within the social network are asked about specific assistance and support they are willing and able to provide (see Figure 9-3) as well as the degree of training they seem willing and able to accept.

All of the above information should be assessed in the person's home, if possible. Barriers to independent living are often obvious in the home and are not considered within a facility setting. Examples abound:

• The MS or stroke victim who faithfully undergoes rehabilitation in the hospital until they can walk 40 steps with a walker, on a tile floor—only to become immobilized at the first step on the carpeting at home;

Activities of Daily Living	Needed		If Needed			Recommendations (Cross-check to Plan of Care)
	No	Yes	Willing but Needs Training	Willing if There Is Respite	Not Able (Reason)	
Mobility						
Transferring						
Walking (ambulation)						
Wheeling						
Personal care						
Bathing						
Dressing						

Fig. 9-3. Excerpt from care assessment record involving the assistance/support the family or significant other is willing and able to provide. The provider should cross-check to ADLs and include as part of the plan of care.

• The patient with Parkinson's disease and related severe muscle weakness who can get out of a hospital bed alone but cannot transfer at home because the bed is too low and lacks a side rail to grasp for leverage;

• The patient with heart disease recovering from a broken hip at home whose neighbors bring hot meals daily with high salt content;

• The patient who is ordered to have six small meals per day but receives meals-on-wheels twice daily and has no way to divide them into appropriate portions;

• The patient who sleeps most of the day as well as at night, gradually weakening because medications are not adjusted downward to mitigate soporific side effects and bed-rest deconditioning secondary to steadily decreasing activity;

• The grieving patient who displays severe memory loss presenting as senile dementia when what is needed is therapy to deal with loss plus social interaction and systematic memory help.

All the information needed does not have to be gathered at the face-to-face interview. The assessment process is augmented by the physician summary, a brief description by the primary physician of conditions under medical management, management regimen, residual problems, relevant laboratory data, precautions, and short- and long-term goals. Just as delivery of medical care is incomplete without knowledge of the social and environmental needs of the client, so it is irresponsible to the person with chronic disabilities to make judgments about service needs without knowledge of medical conditions and their current management.

In addition, if the assessment team finds cause, an in-depth psychological evaluation can be requested. The underlying questions always exist—How is this problem(s) affecting the patient's life? What are the functional implications?

All this information plus the client's self-report complete the basic data base, providing the raw material on which a plan of care can be built *in cooperation* with the patient, the family network, and the full spectrum of care providers.

(NOTE: The terms patient and client have been used interchangeably throughout SCS. We must focus on the person who is seeking help and not allow ourselves to be trapped or confused by the labels that we or others place on this person.)

Data Integration—The Problem-Oriented Record

The assessment provides information. It is important information—but by itself it is not useful. It must be integrated across functional, medical, psychosocial, and environmental aspects of the person's life to identify problems and potential solutions.

The assessment instrument is cross-referenced to support easy correlating of material. Where two areas are particularly related, each is cross-referenced. However, once all data are assembled, the difficult job must be done of analyzing the material and recording it in an easily understood and manageable form. *The problem-oriented record (POR) facilitates the analytic process by which data, dis-*

crete pieces of information, are reorganized into defined problems requiring solution. Once the problem(s) is identified, a plan of care complete with action steps to reach specific goals can be developed and monitored.

In a good record, problems are clearly described, the information supporting the problem definition is clear and identifiable, the actions to be taken to deal with the problem are also clear, and those actions are related to goals set within a time frame to facilitate followup and monitoring. Such a record can be audited, and another caregiver can pick it up and assure continuity of care. It also becomes a useful teaching tool because it can be reviewed objectively for successes and problems.

The working parts of SCS are modeled on the basic components of the POR, problem list, planning flow sheets, process notes, objective data (listed separately for easy review), and medication directory. This system standardizes *how* data are integrated in order to arrive at decisions about needed care. As new providers replace old (staff turnover, vacations, etc.) there is a logical record of how decisions were arrived at, a record that can then be built upon. In the care of the elderly, because of the multiple chronic degenerative problems and their ever-changing functional impact, it is often difficult to determine with a standard descriptive record-keeping system the rationale for care or services provided earlier. With SCS the record becomes a tool that can be used quickly by any provider or caregiver to identify the current problems under management by SCS. If needed, a detailed rationale for particular services can be discerned by systematic tracking of a problem number through the chart.[55]

Problem List.   The problem list is the first page of the record and serves as the index to the record. Each problem is given a name and a number, which are reserved for that problem only and never reused. All entries relative to each problem carry that name and number, so that a review of all actions in relation to each problem is simple. The problem list enables computerization of the record and cross-referencing of related problems by problem number, facilitating quality review and utilization review and thus creating an easily audited and checked record.

Planning Flow Sheets.   The entries on this sheet are the action steps, dated relative to each problem. They are numbered and named as on the problem list. The flow sheets facilitate a quick review of action relative to the goals, by problem, with a date for initial action and one for review.

The more dynamic a case, the more useful this part of the record because the care coordinator/manager does not have to wade through lengthy notes or complex analysis to find out what happened. Problem, goal, action, and dates are easy to follow. The index number allows easy reference to the analysis in the process notes if one needs to understand the reasons for any action or set of actions.

Process Notes.   This part of the record is done first because *it provides the analytic framework that leads to definition of the problem*. Each problem definition is tentative until the care manager (any designated member of the rehabilitation team) has analyzed the supporting information across all relevant aspects of function and is fairly confident as to what the problem is.

It is important to recall that the focus of service management is to maximize function. Therefore the object in defining a functional problem is to ask what difference it makes in the person's life. The question is—So what? If it makes no difference, it probably needs no action.

A simple example makes this focus clear. If a person cannot see well and the medical problem is the specific vision impairment (e.g., cataracts, myopia, etc.), the functional problems could be, say, inability to read, or restricted mobility, or restricted socialization; once this person has glasses that correct the vision impairment, a great many problems are resolved. But if the person had an uncorrected vision problem because of an inability (real or perceived) to afford the glasses, the physician's prescription will remain unfilled until the financial problem is resolved—Solving the functional problems that are secondary to the medical problems depends on resolving the financial problem.

Such an example is deceptively simple. Teasing out the functional problem and relating it appropriately to medical, psychosocial, and environmental factors is usually a complex process.

The process is further complicated by the styles of each profession. Nurses (and physicians) tend to review a patient by body system. Such review pinpoints medical problems but makes it hard (though not impossible) to see how the person's life is affected. A review of the same problem list first by body system and then by function shows how a functional list that considers medical problems as they relate to function can refocus a plan of care (see lists 1 and 2, Circle of Care).

Analysis. SOAP—the analytic process used to organize the data and the analysis of data—begins with the client's view of the situation.

S stands for *subjective*—the patient's description. Patients are the ultimate experts on how they feel and what is being experienced. The use of subjective does not imply that the client's feelings are not real, only that what the client experiences is being discussed.

O stands for *objective*—verified findings from clinical or laboratory tests (listed separately for easy retrieval).

A stands for *assessment meaning analysis.* Given all the information that has been gathered, where does it lead? *What is the problem?* At this point the problem has a name and can be numbered and entered in the problem list.

P stands for the *plan of care.* The actions for chronic patients always fall into two categories. First, what does the person and/or the family have to know to take maximum responsibility for care? This involves client education, family education, and possibly training if there are identified services that patient and family are willing and able to carry out. Second and complementary to client and family education and service mobilization are the formal services required. These may need to include regular respite for caretakers who bear the lion's share of responsibility for care. It sometimes means providing actual services to the caretaker along with the client services, such as meals-on-wheels, financial counseling, therapy, or counseling to deal with stress or to help the caretaker understand the plight of a loved one (especially for spouses of clients with Alzheimer's disease, where memory, personality and cognition diminish).

Fundamentally, the plan of care must be responsive to the needs of the client. The client is viewed holistically, with function as the prime focus and predictor of services. The client also must be viewed within the context of a system—the family and community that share informally and formally in service and care.

The initial assessment and SOAP process are time-consuming, but they provide the service manager with a firm foundation from which to define problems, monitor progress, change services as conditions change, and terminate services no longer needed. Further, the chart with its integrated problem list and plan, when shared appropriately with physician or other caretakers, educates the community of providers to the need for a shared enterprise on behalf of impaired clients. Everyone can come to realize that they cannot and need not operate alone if chronic problems are to be managed.

Medications.   The medications record is virtually a chart within a chart. It is pulled out of the assessment and made a part of the client's ongoing chart. It allows an examination of the interactions between medications as well as interactions with food. (For example, eating licorice when taking digitalis is contraindicated.) Gathering the complete medications record and sharing it with the physician, with the client's consent, can lead to dealing with overmedication and even some underlying problems, often for the first time.

Service Coordination Action Log.   Because SCS was a demonstration project and the first step to eventual statewide implementation, the SCS plan of care goes several steps beyond normal charting. The service management team was asked to develop an ideal plan of care, then to enter in the chart what actually could be delivered. The providers were then asked for an analysis of the reasons for the difference between actual and ideal plans. The reasons that needed services cannot be delivered are information relevant to policy and rarely available to decision-makers.

To facilitate easy notations of barriers encountered when implementing the plan, we developed the action log for the service manager's use as a record of barriers by problem. This log functions as a vital part of regular chart review because it fosters mutual help among staff in dealing with and overcoming barriers to appropriate care.

The POR as a Teaching Tool

A chart review should be held regularly for all staff involved in the evaluation process. At that time new cases are reviewed—assessment data are summarized, problems are listed by function in light of medical and social problems, and actions in the plan of care are reviewed. The training by consultants established a model for constructive critique of the record. Shared experience about real problems to which innovative solutions must be sought creates an environment conducive to self-assessment, staff development, and growth. It also creates an environment in which diverse viewpoints across professional differences can be appreciated.

The record becomes the source of data that can be tracked by individual client, cross-tabulated to develop profiles of client characteristics with service need, and collected for planning purposes. It keeps the system accountable to clients, because services must be arranged acceptable to and, at least in part, implemented by them; to providers, who share in the care of each client; and to payers public and private, whose fiscal support enables care.

Training and Implementation

To implement SCS, initial training for the assessment team composed of rehabilitation nurse or PT/OT and social worker can be done in approximately 48 hours. The initial 24 hours (3 days) provides a theoretical foundation plus experience with the assessment and charting process. After the staff have gained actual field experience in assessment and service management, followup training for 8 to 16 hours is provided. Additional problem-solving sessions of 8 to 16 hours should be offered as part of a staff development process. The SCS coordinator builds from this training through weekly or bimonthly chart reviews and problem-solving sessions as a means of ongoing in-service training.

The instruments discussed earlier were used as basic curriculum materials in the original program. Each staff person received two notebooks. Volume I included the screening and assessment instruments and the POR format with detailed instructions for its proper use.

Two case studies were used to introduce the processes of assessment and of integration and analysis of data, leading to a plan of care. An assessment was demonstrated on film, and the staff analyzed what they had heard and attempted to formulate a functional problem list. A second case study presented assessment data in an organized form, and staff formulated the functional problem list and plan of care.

Volume II was a service manual. It included a description of the system, a section on reimbursement, with special emphasis on Titles XVIII, XIX, and XX of the Social Security Act, and on OAA funds, and descriptions of three simple conceptual tools that helped communicate the meaning of the service delivery system: the circle of care, the health team and its composition, and a chart of the continuum of care/services for the elderly.

The chart illustrating the continuum of care was divided into 10 columns; it functioned as the index for the service manual. A survey was made of all the providers in the five-county area of the demonstration project. Each section of the notebook, correlated to a column of the chart, contained descriptions of the service providers that fit the particular category. Thus there was a concrete way to talk about the range of services and types of providers. It supported discussion of the essential interaction among medical, social, and environmental services (income, housing, transportation) and the role of client, family, social supports, and the service management team in building an appropriate minisystem of care for each client.

MODEL APPROACH FOR PHYSICAL THERAPY EVALUATION OF THE DISABLED ELDERLY

When the initial evaluation by the rehabilitation team results in a referral to physical therapy, the goal of the physical therapy evaluation is to develop a detailed description of the functional losses. Given a description of the ADL tasks affected, the amount of physical and mechanical assistance needed, and the time needed to perform the complete task, it is then possible to study the component factors of the impaired functional skills (range of motion, coordination, strength, proprioception, sensation, balance, posture, etc.). The final treatment plan will use physical therapy procedures chosen to achieve improvement in the total function of the patient.

The ADL assessment developed by Edith Buchwald-Lawton is ideally suited for the initial review of ADL losses or dysfunction because of its precision in evaluation, its reproducibility and reliability as a testing tool, and the low cost of its implementation and utilization.[56] The Lawton ADL evaluation is ideally suited to the evaluation required for the aged because it can measure very small increments of progress. The Lawton assessment has evolved from years of testing and is a precision tool for the evaluation of ADL. The form is divided into an initial summary, 47 indoor ADL tasks, 44 ADL tasks related to mobility in the home and the community, equipment inventory, discharge summary, and a home situation checklist for barriers to independence.

The initial summary provides a description of the basic demographics about the patient with a functional emphasis (time in bed or wheelchair per day, ADL-related equipment owned, patient goals, means of communication, etc.). The initial summary provides an overview, but the core of the assessment is the systematic review of the 91 ADL tasks (fewer as ability allows), with the description of the grade of physical help required to perform a task, the time needed, and, as called for, the distance or number of steps and the height of stairs or curbs. The 91

| One or any combination of the following options is applicable: | |
Grade: I Lifting	Grade: A Assistance
Patient can perform 1–25% of an activity; helper supports/moves 25–99% of patient's body weight	Patient can perform 25–99% of an activity; helper moves/supports 1–25% of patient's body weight
a. Patient cannot maintain sitting balance while moving arms and/or placing legs	a. Patient can maintain sitting balance while using arms to start placing legs and/or wheelchair and its parts.
b. Can place hands but cannot shift sufficient weight on them to move body in any direction.	b. Can shift sufficient weight to hands to move body in necessary direction, by rocking forward and back or from side to side; *Helper* has to steady, move, and guide patient to complete transfer and handle legs/or wheelchair and/or its parts.
c. If a sliding board is used and patient has to be positioned on it and moved across it to complete the transfer and cannot use arms at all, the *grade is L*	*Helper* starts moving patient, who completes transfers
	c. Patient can position self on board if helper slides it halfway under patient, who completes transfer without help, or needs help as in *b*
	d. Patient can perform some but not all motions to place wheelchair and/or parts

Fig. 9-4. Excerpt from Part I of the Lawton ADL evaluation. G, grade; T, time. L indicates an activity involving lifting. (Courtesy of Dr. Edith Lawton.)

tasks are each broken down, and it is presumed that the client will perform the task in both directions as it applies (e.g., into bed from wheelchair and out of bed to wheelchair).

The grades of physical assistance are lifting (L), performing for patient (P), assistance (A), supervision (S), independent (I), not pertinent (X), not feasible at present (O), and not tested or patient refused (N). The grading of physical assistance has been defined on the same model as traditional muscle testing (see Figure 9-4). For a specific grade it is clear to the therapist what quantity of help must be required (100 percent, 75 percent, etc.).

In addition to the grade for physical assistance, the time required to perform the ADL task is also measured. The time to complete a task requires the inclusion of all activities done by the patient and the helper/assistant. The sequence of motions for a particular task are identified, so that it is clear when to start timing, when to finish, and what to include (see Figure 9-5). Time is the only measure of minor improvement currently available, since it measures the patient's coordination/organization of the performance of the ADL task. For the aging patient use of both grade (physical assistance) and time allows documentation of small increments of progress and can also function as positive feedback to the patient when visible progress is slow.

The Lawton assessment also lists any equipment that the patient uses to achieve maximal independence in each ADL task. The description of how the patient achieves maximum independence (physical assistance, time, equipment) can be of great help to nursing staff and the family to ensure followthrough of the training conditions required for independence (e.g., patient requires supervision to transfer wheelchair to toilet but can accomplish it only in a wheelchair with swing away leg rests, with a grab bar to the left of the toilet, wearing glasses, and with Velcro adaptation for trousers). The charting format allows multiple assessments to be recorded on one page, thereby facilitating its use by aides and family for daily care as well as noting progress (Figure 9-6). From the flow chart of ADL tasks an inventory is generated of equipment currently in use, any equipment that will be needed upon discharge, what has been ordered, and what has been received. The rehabilitation team can use this form to assure accurate acquisition of assistive devices needed at discharge; at all times it is possible in 1 or 2 minutes to

Bed to wheelchair	Start Time	Sitting in bed
		Placing wheelchair, removing parts, locking brakes, placing necessary equipment, replacing wheelchair parts
	Finish	Sit in wheelchair, all parts replaced, feet on footrests
	NOTE:	*If helper has to place wheelchair, include in time and grade*
Wheelchair to bed	Start Time	Sitting in wheelchair near bed, feet on footrests
		Placing wheelchair, removing parts, locking brakes; transfer, placing legs, replacing wheelchair parts
	Finish	Sit on bed

Fig. 9-5. An example of timing in the Lawton ADL evaluation. (Courtesy of Dr. Edith Lawton.)

Patient:	Date: Sign:			Date Sign:		
	G	T	Equipment	G	T	Equipment
1 *BED:* Rolling over (L)						
2 Sitting up and reverse (L)						
3 Using signal bell						
4 Using telephone						
5 Bladder care (L)						
6 Bowel care (L)						
7 To commode chair (L)						
8 Reverse (L)						
9 *WHEELCHAIR TO:* Bed (L)						
10 Reverse						
11 Sink (wash and dry hands)						
12 Toilet (L)						
13 Shower (L)						
14 Tub (L)						
15 Car–taxi (L)						
16 Reverse						
17 Placing wheelchair into car (L)						
18 Reverse (L)						

Fig. 9-6. Examples of grading activities involving gross body motions. This excerpt involves transfer from bed to wheelchair. (Courtesy of Dr. Edith Lawton.)

identify any outstanding or missing pieces of equipment essential for independent action.

The validity and relevance of any assessment tool is determined in the day-to-day utilization with patients. The Lawton form has been found to be realistic in design, layout, and length of time needed to maintain it. Its development was facilitated by practitioner criticism. The effectiveness of the Lawton ADL instrument was tested formally in a study by Willard. The goal was to examine reproducibility and reliability—agreement between the grades given by different therapists who evaluated the same patients for physical assistance, time, and equipment. The instrument was found to have high reliability in this regard. For example, for different therapists using the "wheelchair mobility" segment of the form there was 94 percent agreement in evaluation. The high percentage of agreement means that evaluation should consistently show high reproducibility from tester to tester, ensuring effective communication among practitioners.

The Lawton ADL Test is ideal for functional testing and as a base for generating a *physical therapy treatment plan*. The tester needs 6 to 8 hours of orientation to the form. The Lawton ADL test allows organization of large quantities of data, and several assessments can be recorded on a single page. The form is concise, and the flow chart format allows quick scanning of previous and current status. The strongest argument for the use of this form, as opposed to individual practitioners attempting to design their own forms, is that it has been tested for reliability and validity. The Lawton instrument, used as a starting point for planning physical therapy care of the aged, promotes humane care for a fragile population because it can measure small increments of improvement. It thus increases the motivation of the patient to work hard at increasing function. Evaluation must consider patient age, disabilities, and cause of those disabilities as well as emotional needs. The Lawton ADL test is designed to provide a testing environment and approach that considers the unique abilities and needs of the elderly. It is constructed to allow the amount of detail necessary to effectively evaluate and monitor the *slow* but *possible* progress as the elderly go through a process of rehabilitation.

REFERENCES

1. Commission on Chronic Illness: Chronic Illness in the United States, Vol 4, Chronic Illness in a Large City, The Baltimore Study. Harvard University Press, Cambridge, Mass., 1975.
2. Sherwood S: Long term care issues, perspectives and directions. In: Long Term Care: A Handbook for Researchers, Planners and Providers, ed. Sherwood S. Spectrum, New York, 1975, p. 3.
3. Rhode Island Health Services Research, Inc. (SEARCH): Profiles from the Health Statistics Center. Series 4, No. 1, Results of the 1972 and 1975 Health Interview Surveys, 1977.
4. Lawton EB: ADL: Activities of Daily Living Test, A New Form. Rehabilitation Monograph No. 57, Institute of Rehabilitation Medicine, New York University Medical Center, New York, 1979.
5. Aniansson A: Muscle function in old age with special reference to muscle morphology, effect of training and capacity in daily living. Thesis, Departments of Rehabilitation Medicine and Geriatric and Long-Term Care Medicine, University of Goteborg, Sweden, 1980.
6. Jette AM, Branch LG: The Framingham Disability Study: II. Physical Disability among the Aging. Am J Public Health 71:No. 11, 1981.
7. Branch LG: Understanding the Health and Social Service Needs of People over Age 65. Center for Survey Research of the University of Massachusetts and the Joint Center for Urban Studies of MIT and Harvard University, Cambridge, Mass., 1977.
8. Aniansson A, Rundgren A, Sperling L: Evaluation of Functional Capacity in Activities of Daily Living in 70-Year-Old Men and Women. Scand J Rehabil Med 12(4):145–154, 1980.
9. Hook O, Nordquist D, Magnussen K, Sjovall E: Teknik for aldringar. Styrelsen for teknisk utveckling, Utredning 27, Stockholm, 1975.
10. Sperling, L: Evaluation of Upper Extremity Function in 70 Year Old Men and Women. Scand J Rehabil Med 12(4):139–144, 1980.
11. Donnelly RJ: A study of the dynamometer strength of adult males ages 30 to 79. Doctoral dissertation, University of Michigan, Ann Arbor, University of Michigan Microfilm, #1664, 1953.
12. Burke WE, Tuttle WW, Thompson CW, Janney CD, Weber RJ: The relation of grip strength and grip strength endurance to age. J Appl Physiol 5:628, 1953.
13. Asmussen E, Heeboll-Nielsen K: Isometric strength of adult men and women. Communications from the Testing and Observation Institute of the Danish National Association for Infantile Paralysis, vol. 11, 1961.
14. Carroll D: A quantitative test of upper extremity function. J Chronic Dis 18:479, 1965.

15. Petrofsky JS, Lind AR: Isometric strength, endurance and the blood pressure and heart rate responses during isometric exercise in healthy men and women with special reference to age and body fat content. Pfluegers Arch 360:49, 1975.
16. Lautso, K: Jalankulkuliikennie, ominaisuuksia ja teoriaa. Liikennetekniikka OY, Helsinki, 1971.
17. Ayalon A, von Gheluwe B: A comparison study of some mechanical variables from daily life activities in elderly and young people. In: Physical Exercise and Activities for the Ageing. Proceedings of an International Seminar. Wingate Institute of Physical Education and Sport, 1975.
18. Peszcynski M: Senile Gait. Restorative Medicine in Geriatrics. Charles C Thomas, Springfield, Ill., 1963.
19. Hasselkus BR, Shambes GM: Aging and postural sway in women. J Gerontol 30:661, 1975.
20. Azar GJ, Lawton AH: Gait and stepping as factors in the frequent falls of elderly women. Gerontologist 4:83, 1964.
21. Rosow I, Breslau H: A Guttman health scale for the aged. Gerontologist 21:556, 1966.
22. Shanas E: Self-assessment of physical function: White and black elderly of the United States. In: Second Conference on the Epidemiology of Aging. U.S. Department of Health and Human Services, ed. Haynes SG, et al. NIH Pub. No. 80-969, Bethseda, 1980.
23. Uhlenberg P: Changing structure of the older population of the United States of America during the twentieth century. Gerontologist 17:197, 1977.
24. Barry J: Pro/con: Rehabilitation of the aging. J Rehabil 46:3, 1980(b).
25. Benedict RC, Ganikos ML: Coming to terms with ageism in rehabilitation. J Rehabil 47:4, 1981.
26. Blake R: Disabled older persons: A demographic analysis. J Rehabil 47:4, 1981.
27. Independent Living Research Utilization Project: Source Book. Texas Institute for Rehabilitation and Research, 1978.
28. United States Department of Health Education and Welfare: New Facts About Older Americans. Administration on Aging. U.S. Government Printing Office, Washington, D.C., 1973.
29. The Urban Institute: Report of the Comprehensive Service Needs Study. Department of Health, Education and Welfare, Office of Human Development, Rehabilitation Services Administration, Washington, D.C., 1975.
30. Nagi S: An Epidemiology of Adult Disability in the U.S. Mershon Center, Ohio State University, 1975.
31. Rehabilitation Brief, Independent Living Rehabilitation: Results of Five Demonstration projects. National Institute of Handicapped Research, Washington, D.C., 1979.
32. Driscoll J, Marquis B, Corcoran P, Fay F: Second generation: New England. Am Rehabil 3:6, 1978.
33. Reid DW, Ziegler M: A desired control measure for studying the psychological adjustment of the elderly. Paper presented at the symposium on Goal-Specific Locus of Control Scale—A New Step in I-E Research held at the meeting of the American Psychology Association, Toronto, Sep 1978.
34. Boll TJ: A rationale for neuropsychological evaluation. Prof Psychol 8:64, 1977.
35. Center for the Study of Aging and Human Development: Multidimensional Functional Assessment: The OARS Methodology. 2nd ed. Duke University Medical Center, Durham, N.C., 1978.
36. Fortinsky RH, Granger CV, Seltzer GB: The use of functional assessment in understanding home care needs. Med Care 19:5, 1981.

37. Stewart CPU: A prediction score for geriatric rehabilitation prospects. Rheumatol Rehabil 19:239, 1980.
38. Kahn RL, Goldberg AI: The relationship of mental and physical status in institutionalized aged persons. Am J Psychol 117:120, 1960.
39. Magid S, Hearn CR: Characteristics of geriatric patients as related to nursing needs. J Nurs Studies 18:2, 1981.
40. Adler MK, Brown CC, Acton P: Stroke rehabilitation—Is age a determinant? J Am Geriatr Soc 28:11, 1980.
41. Hall MRP: The assessment of disability in the geriatric patient. Rheumatol Rehabil 15, 1976.
42. Carroll D: Proceedings of a Symposium on the Motivation of the Physically Disabled. ed Nichols, PJR, 1968.
43. Report by the Comptroller General to the Congress: Entering a Nursing Home—Costly Implications for Medicaid and the Elderly. U.S. Government Printing Office, Washington, D.C., PAD-80-12, Nov 29, 1979.
44. Currie CT, Moore JT, Friedmen SW, Warshaw GA: Assessment of elderly patients at home: Report of 50 cases. J Am Geriatr Soc 29:9, 1981.
45. Tickle LS, Yerxa EJ: Need satisfaction of older persons living in the community and in institutions. Part 2, Role of activity. Am J Occup Ther 35:10, 1981.
46. Developing Comprehensive and Coordinated Service Systems for Older People: Lessons from the Nebraska Demonstration. Project funded by the Administration of Aging, Office of Human Development, Department of Health and Human Services, Grant No. 90-A-1968.
47. Hicks BC, Segal J, Quinn JL, Raisz H: Triage: Coordinated Services to the Elderly. Final Report. National Technical Information Service, Springfield, Va., Pub Order PB-135-824.
48. Future Directions for Aging Policy: A Human Service Model. A Report of the Select Committee on Aging, U.S. House of Representatives, Ninety-sixth Congress. Comm. Publ. No. 96-226. U.S. Government Printing Office, Washington, D.C., May 1980.
49. Katz S, Ford AB, Moskowitz RW, et al: Studies of illness in the aged. JAMA 185:914, 1963.
50. Akpom C, Katz S: Index of ADL. Med Care 14:116, 1976.
51. Falcone AR: Long-Term Care Information System Assessment Process. Funded by W.K. Kellogg Foundation, Battle Creek, Mich., Grant 5000.
52. Lawton MP, Brody EM: Assessment of older people: Self-maintaining and instrumental activities of daily living. Gerontologist 9:179, 1969.
53. Densen PM: Patients Classification for Long-Term Care: User's Manual. DHEW Pub. No. (HRA) 74-3107, Health Resources Administration, Bureau of Health Services Research and Evaluation, Washington, D.C.
54. Buchwald-Lawton E: Activities of Daily Living. McGraw-Hill, New York, 1963.
55. Weed LL: Medical Records, Medical Evaluation and Patient Care. Case Western Reserve University Press, Cleveland, 1971.
56. Buchwald-Lawton E: ADL—Activities of Daily Living: A New Form. New York University Medical Center, Institute of Rehabilitation Medicine, New York, 1979.

Index

Page numbers followed by f indicate figures; page numbers followed by t indicate tables